The Irving B. Harris Award of the ZERO TO THREE Press

IRENE CHATOOR is the winner of an Irving B. Harris Award of the ZERO TO THREE Press. Created by the late Irving B. Harris, these generous stipends offered essential support to outstanding authors for the development of book manuscripts that address issues of emerging importance to the multidisciplinary infant–family field. The ZERO TO THREE Press Editorial Board selected the recipients from among manuscripts submitted for consideration during five competitions. *Diagnosis and Treatment of Feeding Disorders in Infants, Toddlers, and Young Children* is a result of Harris' generosity and belief in the power of books to make a lasting difference in the way we care for infants, toddlers, and families.

DIAGNOSIS AND TREATMENT OF FEEDING DISORDERS

in Infants, Toddlers, and Young Children

IRENE CHATOOR, MD

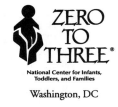

ZERO TO THREE®

National Center for Infants, Toddlers, and Families

Washington, DC

Published by

ZERO TO THREE
2000 M St., NW, Suite 200
Washington, DC 20036-3307
(202) 638-1144; Fax: (202) 638-0851
Toll-free orders (800) 899-4301
Web: http://www.zerotothree.org

The mission of the ZERO TO THREE Press is to publish authoritative research, practical resources, and new ideas for those who work with and care about infants, toddlers, and their families. Books are selected for publication by an independent Editorial Board. The views contained in this book are those of the author and do not necessarily reflect those of ZERO TO THREE: National Center for Infants, Toddlers and Families, Inc.

These materials are intended for education and training to help promote a high standard of care by professionals. Use of these materials is voluntary and their use does not confer any professional credentials or qualification to take any registration, certification, board or licensure examination, and neither confers nor infers competency to perform any related professional functions.

The user of these materials is solely responsible for compliance with all local, state or federal rules, regulations or licensing requirements. Despite efforts to ensure that these materials are consistent with acceptable practices, they are not intended to be used as a compliance guide and are not intended to supplant or to be used as a substitute for or in contravention of any applicable local, state or federal rules, regulations or licensing requirements. ZERO TO THREE expressly disclaims any liability arising from use of these materials in contravention of such rules, regulations or licensing requirements. The views expressed in these materials represent the opinions of the respective authors. Publication of these materials does not constitute an endorsement by ZERO TO THREE of any view expressed herein, and ZERO TO THREE expressly disclaims any liability arising from any inaccuracy or misstatement.

Cover and text design: Design Consultants

Library of Congress Cataloging-in-Publication Data

Chatoor, Irene.
  Diagnosis and treatment of feeding disorders in infants, toddlers, and young children / Irene Chatoor.
    p. ; cm.
  Includes bibliographical references.
  ISBN 978-1-934019-33-7
  1. Eating disorders in children. I. Title.
  [DNLM: 1. Feeding and Eating Disorders of Childhood--diagnosis. 2. Child, Preschool. 3. Failure to Thrive--diagnosis. 4. Failure to Thrive--therapy. 5. Feeding and Eating Disorders of Childhood--therapy. 6. Infant. WM 175 C493d 2009]
  RJ506.E18C43 2009
  618.92'8526--dc22

                              2009005598

10 9 8 7 6 5 4 3 2
ISBN 978-1-934019-33-7
Printed in the United States of America

Suggested citation:
Chatoor, I. (2009). *Diagnosis and treatment of feeding disorders in infants, toddlers, and young children*. Washington, DC: ZERO TO THREE.

DEDICATION

In memory of my parents Maria and Hugo Koch and my husband Ram Chatoor.

Their love has given me direction and their sufferings have taught me compassion.

CONTENTS

ACKNOWLEDGMENTS

THIS BOOK WAS MADE POSSIBLE through more than 20 years of clinical work and research. During this time, I have met many families with infants and young children who have struggled with feeding problems. I want to express my gratitude to these families for sharing their stories with me. Their suffering and trust have challenged me to look beyond what I could find in the literature and made me turn to research. These families have given me as much as I have been able to give to them.

The clinical work and the research on feeding disorders would not have been possible without the collaboration of a wonderful clinical and research team. More than 25 years ago, Benny Kerzner, MD, the chair of gastroenterology at Children's National Medical Center, brought together members from different disciplines including nutrition, occupational therapy, hearing and speech, psychology, and psychiatry. Together we formed a multidisciplinary team for the diagnosis and treatment of feeding disorders. Although team members have come and gone over the years, some have stayed and become the rocks of the team. I want to express my special thanks to Dr. Kerzner for his ongoing collaboration and support, to his nurse practitioner, Laura McWade Paez, and to his nurse clinician, Lori Stern, who both continue to serve as team coordinators today. I also want to express my thanks to occupational therapist, Randy Simensen, who during many years of collaboration has taught me about sensory difficulties. Many thanks to nutritionists Leila Beker, PhD, and Lauren Rhee who have helped me to sort out the nutritional aspects of feeding disorders.

I want to express my gratitude to my research mentor, David Reiss, MD, who has helped me to translate my clinical experiences into research questions. I have enjoyed the collaboration with Jody Ganiban, PhD, who has a background in developmental psychology and with Robert Hirsch, PhD, who has provided his statistical expertise to our studies. I also want to thank my colleagues Joyce Harrison, MD, and Miguel Macaoay, MD, for their participation in our clinical work and research, and social workers Sue Besherov, Kathy Connell, Marianne Katz, and Valerie Truett for their contribution to the research on Infantile Anorexia. Finally, I want to thank my research assistants Jaclyn Shepard, Amy Hahn, and Laura Brinkmeier for their tireless work; and Amy and Laura in particular for their invaluable editorial support.

INTRODUCTION

FOR MOST INFANTS, feeding appears to be a natural process. However, approximately 25% of otherwise normally developing infants and up to 80% of those with developmental handicaps have been reported to have feeding problems. In addition, 1% to 2% of infants have been found to have serious feeding difficulties associated with poor weight gain. Feeding disorders not only disrupt the infant's early development but have been linked to later deficits in cognitive development, behavioral problems, as well as anxiety disorders and eating disorders during childhood, adolescence, and young adulthood. Consequently, it is extremely important to identify, understand, and treat early feeding problems.

In the past, the term *failure to thrive* (FTT) was used as a catchall diagnosis for all feeding disorders. Clinicians initially distinguished between two forms of FTT: organic FTT and nonorganic FTT. Organic FTT represents growth failure that can be traced to a medical cause. Nonorganic FTT is thought to reflect maternal deprivation or parental psychopathology. A third category was later added to describe growth failure that is related to a mixture of organic and environmental factors. In recent years, the use of FTT as a diagnostic category for feeding disorders has been sharply criticized. A primary concern is that not all infants with feeding disorders demonstrate growth failure (i.e., FTT). Consistent with this view, some researchers have argued that FTT represents a symptom rather than a diagnostic category.

To address the need for diagnostic criteria for feeding disorders, the American Psychiatric Association (1994) adopted a descriptive approach in the *Diagnostic and Statistical Manual of Mental Disorders* (4th ed.; *DSM–IV*) and introduced "Feeding Disorder of Infancy and

Early Childhood" as a diagnostic category. The specific criteria include (a) feeding disturbance as manifested by persistent failure to eat adequately with significant failure to gain weight or significant loss of weight over at least 1 month, (b) the disturbance is not due to an associated gastrointestinal or other medical condition, (c) the condition is not better accounted for by another mental disorder (e.g., Rumination Disorder) or by lack of available food, (d) the onset is before age 6 years. However, the diagnostic criteria in *DSM–IV* exclude whole groups of children who have feeding disorders without weight problems, and feeding disorders associated with medical conditions. To address this problem, some authors have suggested subclassification systems of feeding disorders with various organic and nonorganic causes or have used a multidimensional approach, combining descriptive and etiological categories. However, there has been little uniformity in terms, and because of vague definitions of symptoms, confusion continues among clinicians and researchers regarding what constitutes a feeding disorder. Different diagnostic labels have been used to describe overlapping symptomatology, and the same label has been used to describe different feeding problems. In addition to the confusing use of labels to describe various feeding and growth problems, most of the reports only describe some clinical symptoms but fail to characterize how the described feeding disorder can be differentiated from other feeding disorders and from more transient or subclinical feeding problems. Differences in the description and labeling of feeding disorders have also caused confusion over how to treat children with these disorders.

To address the question of how to differentiate various severe feeding problems from each other and from transient or milder feeding difficulties, I have developed a classification system that describes the phenomenology and provides operational diagnostic criteria for six subtypes of feeding disorders in infants and young children. The original criteria (Chatoor, 2002) were modified with the help of the Task Force for Research Diagnostic Criteria for Infants and Preschool Children (Scheeringa et al., 2003), and were further developed with the help of a national work group of early childhood specialists in the field of psychiatry and psychology. These efforts were supported by the American Academy of Child Psychiatry and the American Psychiatric Association. The diagnostic criteria for the six feeding disorders were included in *Diagnostic Classification of Mental Health and Developmental Disorders of Infancy and Early Childhood: Revised Edition—DC:0–3R* (ZERO TO THREE, 2005) and recently explained in the chapter "A Classification of Feeding Disorders of Infancy and Early Childhood" (Chatoor & Ammaniti, 2007) in *Age and Gender Considerations in Psychiatric Diagnosis: A Research Agenda for DSM-V* (Narrow, First, Sirovatka, & Regier, 2007) published by the American Psychiatric Press.

The diagnostic criteria for the six feeding disorders described in this book include clinical symptoms that differentiate one feeding disorder from another and measures of impairment that differentiate feeding disorders from less severe subclinical feeding problems. The areas of impairment primarily concern nutrition—for example, growth failure, specific dietary deficiencies, or inadequate food intake threatening the child's health and growth—but also include delays in oral motor and speech development, and separation and social anxiety, particularly in cases of Sensory Food Aversions. Although the six subtypes of feeding disorders show some overlapping symptoms and some overlapping criteria for impairment, they represent different combinations of symptoms and different areas of impairment that are believed to be related to different etiologies.

This classification of six subtypes of feeding disorders is not all-inclusive but covers the most commonly seen feeding disorders associated with behavioral symptoms. There are other severe feeding disorders, such as those associated with neurological conditions (e.g., cerebral palsy) or with anatomical defects of the oropharynx (e.g., cleft lip or palate). However, these feeding disorders are usually managed by professionals from occupational therapy and other disciplines.

I will begin this book with a description of the developmental progression of feeding during infancy and early childhood, and a discussion of child and parent characteristics that can disrupt feeding. Then I will present the first four feeding disorders in sequence according to the developmental stage at which they arise, followed by the last two disorders, Posttraumatic Feeding Disorder and Feeding Disorder Associated With a Concurrent Medical Condition, which can arise at any age of the child.

The first feeding disorder described is Feeding Disorder of State Regulation, which is seen in young infants during the first few months of life. It is followed by Feeding Disorder of Caregiver–Infant Reciprocity. This feeding disorder has drawn much research attention and has mostly been described as nonorganic FTT (NOFTT) or as maternal deprivation or neglect. I chose this new description because the main problem seems to lie in the mother's inability to connect with her infant, and labels such as maternal deprivation or neglect have a mother-blaming quality that further interferes with reaching out to these mothers.

The next two chapters discuss Infantile Anorexia and Sensory Food Aversions. These are the most common feeding disorders that have been referred to the Multidisciplinary Feeding Disorders Clinic at Children's National Medical Center. Both feeding disorders become evident during the first 3 years of life, when young children are transitioned to self-feeding, and when issues of autonomy and dependency have to be negotiated between parents and child. In the chapter on Infantile Anorexia, I describe in detail how parents can facilitate internal regulation of eating and self-calming in the young child. This intervention is critical for children with Infantile Anorexia but is important for all children and should be part of the treatment of all feeding disorders.

Each chapter is organized to start with the *nosology*, a description of the terms that have been used by other authors to describe some symptoms of this specific feeding disorder, followed by the diagnostic criteria, the clinical presentation, course, etiology, and treatment. In each chapter, I will discuss research findings and add my clinical experience. All chapters have case presentations to illustrate specific diagnostic and treatment issues. The final chapter will address the comorbidity of two or three feeding disorders. These complex feeding disorders are a special challenge for the clinician, and it is critical to diagnose and treat each feeding disorder in order for the intervention to be successful.

To direct the reader to a particular chapter in the book according to specific feeding problems of the child, I have included a table showing the most common complaints and associated disorders (p. 4). Because food refusal is the most common feeding problem associated with feeding disorders, I have also included a table that clarifies the different types of food refusal that can be seen in infants and young children, and what diagnoses are associated with different types of food refusal (p. 5). It is my hope that that this book can serve as a practical guide for practitioners in the field and be a stimulant for further research.

References

American Psychiatric Association. (1994). *Diagnostic and statistical manual of mental disorders* (4th ed.). Washington, DC: Author.

Chatoor, I. (2002). Feeding disorders in infants and toddlers: Diagnosis and treatment. *Child and Adolescent Psychiatric Clinics of North America, 11*, 163–183.

Chatoor, I., & Ammaniti, M. (2007). A classification of feeding disorders of infancy and early childhood. In W. E. Narrow, M. B. First, P. Sirovatka, & D. A. Regier (Eds.), *Age and gender considerations in psychiatric diagnosis: A research agenda for DSM-V* (pp. 227–242). Arlington, VA: American Psychiatric Press.

Narrow, W. E., First, M. B., Sirovatka, P., & Regier, D. A. (Eds.). (2007). *Age and gender considerations in psychiatric diagnosis: A research agenda for DSM-V*. Arlington, VA: American Psychiatric Press.

Scheeringa, M., Anders, T., Boris, N., Carter, A., Chatoor, I., Egger, H., et al. (2003). Research diagnostic criteria for infants and preschool children: The process and empirical support. *Journal of the American Academy of Child and Adolescent Psychiatry, 42*, 1504–1512.

ZERO TO THREE (2005). *Diagnostic classification of mental health and developmental disorders of infancy and early childhood: Revised edition (DC:0–3R)*. Washington, DC: Author.

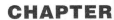

DEVELOPMENT OF REGULATION OF FEEDING AND EMOTIONS

AN IMPORTANT DEVELOPMENTAL PROCESS in the first years of life is the acquisition of autonomous internal regulation of feeding. The infant becomes increasingly aware of his hunger and satiety cues and responds accordingly by communicating his interest to eat when hungry and ceasing to accept food when he feels full. Under ideal conditions, the infant is able to clearly signal his hunger to his caregiver, who in turn, acknowledges the signal and responds by feeding the infant. At the same time, the infant gives clear signals when full and does not accept any more food, and the caregiver stops feeding.

This development of autonomous internal regulation of feeding and emotions unfolds in three stages: (a) state regulation, (b) dyadic reciprocity, and (c) transition to self-feeding and regulation of emotions.

Achieving State Regulation

Whereas in utero the fetus's nutritional demands are met through the maternal umbilical cord, upon birth, infants must actively and clearly signal hunger and satiety to caregivers. During the first few months of life, they must establish both rhythms of sleep and wakefulness, and of feeding and elimination. The infant must signal to the caregiver through crying when hungry and through ceasing to suckle when satiated. Most infants have a distinct cry when hungry, in contrast to other types of cries, such as for pain, fear, or tiredness. Ideally, these distinct cries become increasingly discernable for parents during the first few weeks of life, thereby developing a communication system that allows the infant to express her needs. However, to feed successfully, the infant must also be able to attain a state of calm alertness. If the infant cannot calm herself for feeding, or on the other hand, if she is too sleepy to suckle, the result will be inefficient and stressful feedings for both the infant and parent.

Caregivers must learn to differentiate between the different infant cries and between the infant's hunger and satiety cues and respond appropriately, thus facilitating the infant's internal regulation of feeding. Establishment of the infant–parent communication system is essential to establishing nutritional homeostasis—a state in which the infant's nutritional needs for growth and development are met. However, if parents are challenged by confusing, indiscernible cries, they may respond erroneously by feeding or not feeding their infant. Consequently, the infant's and parents' distinction between hunger and satiety can become confused, which may lead to under- or overfeeding.

Achieving Dyadic Reciprocity

By 2 months, infants develop a social smile and begin to respond in a more active way to their caretakers. Parent and infant interactions become increasingly characterized by mutual eye contact and gazing, reciprocal vocalizations, and mutual physical closeness expressed through touching and cuddling. Reflexive hunger cues decrease, while intentional cues, such as vocalization for food, begin to emerge. A more mature communication pattern evolves as infants begin to regulate caregivers actively and purposefully through their body language and vocalizations. Through receiving stronger and clearer hunger and satiety cues from the infant, caregivers learn to regulate the presentation and withdrawal of food accordingly. Feeding interactions become a mutually regulated process, enjoyable for both infant and caregiver.

However, the mutually regulated processes may not develop or may become derailed when the infant's hunger signals are weak or difficult to read, or when the parents are preoccupied with their own internal needs and unable to tune in to their infant's needs. They may feed their infants sporadically and inefficiently, resulting in inadequate nutrition. Parent and child may not develop a reciprocal relationship, and the infant may be at risk for developing a feeding disorder of failed reciprocity, as will be discussed in chapter 3.

Transition to Self-Feeding and Regulation of Emotions

Between 6 months and 3 years of age, motor and cognitive maturation enable the infant to become physically and emotionally more independent. Autonomy versus dependency has to be negotiated daily during the parent–infant feeding interactions. During each meal, mother and infant need to negotiate who is going to place the spoon in the infant's mouth. As the infant becomes more competent, the parent needs to facilitate the infant's learning to feed himself. During this transition to self-feeding, the infant not only needs to understand the difference between hunger and satiety but also needs to differentiate the physical sensations of hunger and fullness from emotional experiences (e.g., eliciting comfort, affection, feelings of anger or frustration).

For the infant to learn this differentiation, caregivers need to respond differentially to the infant's hunger and satiety cues and affective expressions. This includes offering food when the infant signals hunger, abstaining from offering food when the infant needs affection or calming through tactile sensations, terminating the meal when the infant appears satiated, and not insisting that the infant keeps eating until his plate or jar of baby food is empty. Through the parents' distinct handling of the infant's hunger, satiety, and emotional states, the infant learns by association and begins to differentiate these inner experiences.

Conversely, if the parent misinterprets the infant's emotional cues when she desires physical and emotional comfort by feeding him, the infant may confuse hunger with emotional experiences and associate eating with emotional calming. He then may become conditioned to eat when feeling sad, lonely, or frustrated. External regulation of feeding may evolve based on the emotional experiences of the infant.

Ideally, the infant gives clear, discernable cues, and the parents interpret these signals correctly. If, on the other hand, the infant gives weak hunger cues, this often raises the parents' anxiety and causes confusion. Out of concern for the infant's nutritional needs, the parents may try to override the infant's cues by feeding him, even if the infant is not interested and may refuse to open his mouth. Feeding becomes a highly emotionally charged battleground, pitting the infant's food refusal against the parents' increasing concern about his low volume of food intake. Conversely, if an infant gives weak signals of satiety and is easily comforted by food when distressed, parents may unknowingly be contributing to their child's learning to eat when emotionally distressed or when seeking pleasure.

These early formative years are critical in the development of the child's internal versus external regulation of eating and the differentiation of physiological sensations of hunger and fullness from emotional experiences, such as anger, frustration, and the wish for affection. As described above, maladaptive feeding patterns may emerge during these three developmental stages, if the infant gives poor signals of either hunger or satiety, or the caregiver is unable to interpret the infant's signals correctly and respond accordingly. A feeding disorder may emerge if these feeding patterns become chronic, compromising the infant's growth and development.

The following table illustrates parents' most common concerns about the infant's or toddler's feeding behavior and points to the chapters that address these concerns.

One of the most common parent complaints is the child's food refusals. This behavior can be associated with four different feeding disorders and can be an expression of oppositional behavior in general. The Food Refusal chart (page 5) describes the various types of food refusal and highlights the role of weight in the differential diagnosis.

Chief Complaints and Associated Feeding Disorders

CHIEF COMPLAINT	PROCEED TO CHAPTER:
Has a poor appetite and does not eat enough to grow. Shows little hunger and interest in feeding and wants to play rather than eat.	*If < 6 months old:* Chapter 2: Feeding Disorder of State Regulation *If > 6 months old:* Chapter 4: Infantile Anorexia
Has a limited diet of a few foods. Consistently refuses certain foods or whole food groups.	Chapter 5: Sensory Food Aversions Chapter 6: Posttraumatic Feeding Disorder
Refuses to drink from a bottle or cup, but eats solids. Refuses to eat solid foods, but drinks from a bottle or cup.	Chapter 6: Posttraumatic Feeding Disorder
Refuses all solid foods, but eats pureed foods.	Chapter 5: Sensory Food Aversions Chapter 6: Posttraumatic Feeding Disorder
Refuses most or all feedings and depends on nasogastric/gastrostomy tube feedings.	Chapter 6: Posttraumatic Feeding Disorder Chapter 7: Feeding Disorder Associated With a Concurrent Medical Condition
Refuses to eat something one day, but may eat it the next day.	*If there are no weight concerns:* Oppositional Feeding Behavior which can be associated with food refusal of toddlers in general *If there are weight concerns:* Chapter 4: Infantile Anorexia
Cries a lot and arches during feedings. Tires quickly during feedings and eats too little.	*If < 6 months old:* Chapter 2: Feeding Disorder of State Regulation Chapter 7: Feeding Disorder Associated With a Concurrent Medical Condition
Sleeps through feedings.	*If < 6 months old:* Chapter 2: Feeding Disorder of State Regulation
Gags or vomits before, during, or after feedings.	Chapter 6: Posttraumatic Feeding Disorder Chapter 5: Sensory Food Aversions Chapter 7: Feeding Disorder Associated With a Concurrent Medical Condition
Cries when positioned for feeding or when presented with food.	Chapter 6: Posttraumatic Feeding Disorder

Food Refusal Chart

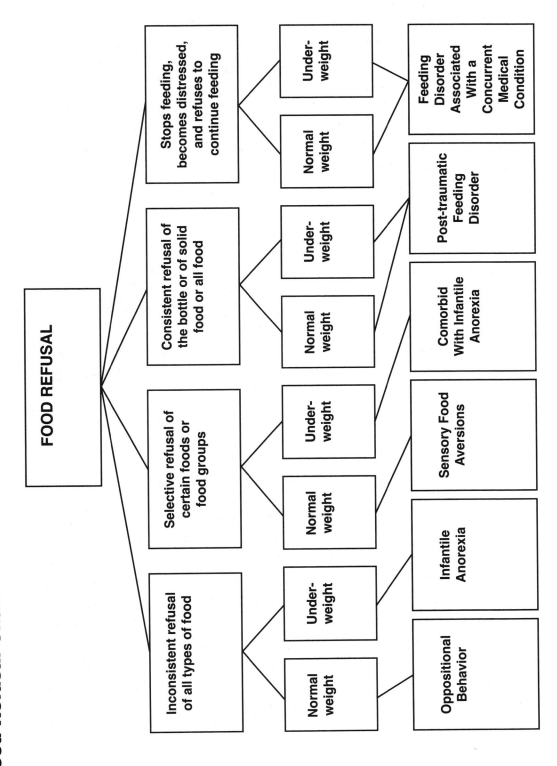

FOOD REFUSAL

- Stops feeding, becomes distressed, and refuses to continue feeding
  - Under-weight
  - Normal weight
  → Feeding Disorder Associated With a Concurrent Medical Condition

- Consistent refusal of the bottle or of solid food or all food
  - Under-weight
  - Normal weight
  → Post-traumatic Feeding Disorder
  → Comorbid With Infantile Anorexia

- Selective refusal of certain foods or food groups
  - Under-weight
  - Normal weight
  → Sensory Food Aversions

- Inconsistent refusal of all types of food
  - Under-weight
  - Normal weight
  → Infantile Anorexia
  → Oppositional Behavior

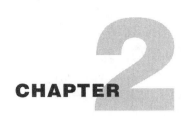

CHAPTER 2

FEEDING DISORDER OF STATE REGULATION

Nosology

IN THE PAST, my colleagues and I have described this feeding disorder as Feeding Disorder of Homeostasis (Chatoor, Dickson, Schaefer, & Egan, 1985; Chatoor et al., 1997) because it usually begins in the postnatal period when infants need to transition from continuous feedings through the umbilical cord and a state of homeostasis in utero, to a new state of homeostasis with established rhythms of sleep and wakefulness and of feeding and elimination. To feed successfully and establish a state of nutritional homeostasis, infants need to reach and maintain a state of calm alertness. However, some infants have difficulties in state regulation; they are too irritable and can't calm themselves in order to initiate or continue feedings, or they are hard to arouse and sleep through feedings. Consequently, I have changed the name of this feeding disorder to Feeding Disorder of State Regulation.

Symptoms of excessive crying and difficulty feeding in young infants are often referred to in the literature as Infant Colic (Miller-Loncar, Bigsby, High, Wallach, & Lester, 2004; Zwart, Vellema-Goud, & Brand, 2007). The emphasis in Infant Colic is on excessive crying, which is usually defined by the Wessel rule of three criteria: crying for 3 or more hours per day, for at least 3 days of the week, for at least 3 weeks (Wessel, Cobb, Jackson, Harris, & Detwil, 1954). Although many studies report on feeding difficulties in Infant Colic, the nature of the feeding difficulties has not been defined. The criteria described below focus on the feeding difficulties of young infants who have difficulty with state regulation and who would be considered by some to have Infant Colic. The criteria for Feeding Disorder of State Regulation were included in *Diagnostic Classification of Mental Health and*

Developmental Disorders of Infancy and Early Childhood: Revised Edition (*DC:0–3R*; ZERO TO THREE, 2005) and were included in Chatoor and Ammaniti's (2007) chapter in *Age and Gender Considerations in Psychiatric Diagnosis: A Research Agenda for DSM-V* (Narrow, First, Sirovatka, & Regier, 2007).

Diagnostic Criteria

A. The infant's feeding difficulties start in the first few months of life and should be present for at least 2 weeks.

B. The infant has difficulty reaching and maintaining a calm state of alertness for feeding; he or she is either too sleepy or too agitated and/or distressed to feed.

C. The infant fails to gain age-appropriate weight or may show loss of weight.

D. The infant's feeding difficulties cannot be explained by a physical illness.

Clinical Presentation

This feeding disorder begins in the postnatal period and is characterized by irregular, poor feedings and inadequate food intake. Infants with this feeding disorder exhibit difficulties in state regulation, which interfere with their ability to feed effectively. They have difficulty reaching and maintaining a state of calm alertness necessary for feeding. Some are too irritable and cry excessively and cannot calm themselves for feeding. Others are too sleepy and cannot wake up or stay awake long enough to feed adequately. The parent is often stressed by the infant's irritability and difficulty feeding and may be anxious or depressed, or both, or may present with more severe psychopathology. Mother–infant interactions during feeding are often characterized by irritability and/or sleepiness of the infant, maternal anxiety and tension, and poor engagement between mother and infant (Chatoor et al., 1997).

The case described below illustrates the feeding difficulties of a young infant who has difficulty calming himself, and the impact this has on the mother–infant relationship during feeding.

Example: Juan was 3 months old when he was admitted to the hospital and referred for a psychiatric evaluation because of his feeding difficulties and "failure to thrive" since birth. A medical workup did not find any organic reason to explain Juan's feeding difficulties and his poor weight gain. Although Juan was born full-term and weighed 7 pounds at birth, he had difficulty drinking from the breast. His mother, Mrs. Avila, said that he had cried a lot from birth and had difficulty calming and latching on to the breast. During feedings he wiggled a lot and often lost the nipple and started to cry, which would then end the feeding. When he was 4 weeks old, Mrs. Avila reluctantly switched him to bottle feedings because he was losing weight. Although his intake improved somewhat on bottle feedings, he gained weight very slowly and was still less than 8 pounds at 3 months. Mrs. Avila appeared tired and described how Juan would drink only 1, 2, or 3 ounces at a time, wiggle and cry, and refuse to continue with the feeding. After a few hours, he might cry again as if he were hungry. However, she could not settle him to feed, and he would continue to cry inconsolably for hours. Mrs. Avila said that she would attempt to feed him an average of 10 to 15 times in a 24-hour period, that Juan would cry a lot during the day and at night, and that everybody in the family was getting very little sleep.

The observation of mother–infant interactions during feeding revealed that Juan was a very alert and wiggly baby who had difficulty settling in his mother's arms. While drinking from the bottle, he would kick his feet and move around with his arms, and soon the nipple of the bottle would slip out of his mouth. This upset him, and he started crying. Mrs. Avila appeared anxious, and tried to restart him by changing his position in various ways, but this only agitated him more. After repeated unsuccessful attempts to continue the feeding, mother and baby appeared exhausted, and Mrs. Avila gave up.

Course of Feeding Disorder

There are no empirical studies that have followed infants with a Feeding Disorder of State Regulation over time to gain a better understanding of what happens to them as they get older. However, there are some interesting follow-up reports from Sweden of infants who were diagnosed with Colic. As explained earlier, Infant Colic focuses on excessive crying, a problem of state regulation, but Colic is often associated with feeding problems. Lindberg, Bohlin, and Hagekull (1991) reported from a large questionnaire study that at 30–70 weeks of age, formerly colicky infants had a worse mood and problems with concentration when fed. A follow-up study of formerly colicky children at 4 years of age by Canivet, Jakobsson, and Hagander (2000) indicated that the children continued to be more emotional, had more temper tantrums, were much less likely than controls to enjoy meals and to like eating, and were more likely to complain of stomach aches. These studies indicate that early problems in regulation of state and feeding may pose some vulnerability for these infants to continue to have eating problems, and further research is needed.

Etiology

There are no empirical studies that have explained why some infants have more difficulty in regulation of state than others and develop feeding problems. However, studies on Infant Colic and feeding problems may shed some light on the etiology of feeding problems related to infants' difficulty in state regulation and feeding. A study of Infant Colic and feeding difficulties by Miller-Loncar and colleagues (2004) found that these infants showed more evidence of reflux; more sucking and feeding problems as evidenced by arrhythmic jaw movements and difficulty coordinating sucking, swallowing, and breathing; less responsiveness during feeding interactions with their mothers; and more episodes of discomfort during feedings. The authors raised the possibility that disorganized feeding patterns in infants with Colic indicate an underlying disorder in behavioral regulation.

A study by Zwart and colleagues (2007) of 104 infants who were hospitalized because of persistent Colic found that 71% of the infants had feeding problems, including poor feeding, regurgitation, and vomiting. Only 2 infants were found to have possible gastro-esophageal reflux, whereas the rest of the infants had no medical problems to explain their crying behavior and feeding difficulties. However, the authors found that the proportion of complicated pregnancies, including preeclampsia, premature labor, vacuum or forceps delivery, or evidence of fetal distress was considerably larger in the Colic group (85%) than in a comparison group (37%). These authors hypothesized that complications during pregnancy and childbirth may predispose parents to be hyperresponsive to their infant's crying behavior. In support of this hypothesis, Zwart and colleagues found that counseling the parents and sending them home from the hospital at night allowed both the infants and parents to settle down and break the cycle of mutual distress. Most infants showed a rapid improvement within 1–2 days to crying, feeding, and sleeping behavior that was considered to be in the normal range.

Treatment

Because there are no empirical data on how to best treat infants with a Feeding Disorder of State Regulation, I have developed an individualized approach to helping these infants and their families. The intervention can be directed toward the infant, toward the mother, and toward the mother–infant interaction. Videotaping the mother and infant during feedings and observing the videotape together with the parents can facilitate a discussion of what triggers the baby's distress and what calms her. If the infant is too sleepy to feed and difficult to arouse, gentle infant massage may stimulate her and help to improve her alertness and facilitate better feeding. If the infant is too irritable and fidgety to feed, reducing stimulation before and during feedings by taking her to a quiet room and swaddling her during feedings may help to settle the infant and facilitate better feedings (McKenzie, 1991). If the mother is exhausted, overly anxious, or depressed, the mother's difficulties have to be addressed for her to be more effective with her infant. However, in cases where the infant tires easily and is unable to take in adequate calories to grow in spite of all efforts to improve the feedings, nasogastric tube feedings may have to be considered to supplement oral feedings.

The case below describes how infant and parent vulnerabilities can interact with each other and lead to severe feeding difficulties. The case illustrates how the intervention for both mother and infant helped to break the cycle of mother–infant distress, facilitate more enjoyable mother–infant interactions, and bring about the infant's healthy feeding development.

Example: Mark was admitted to the hospital at 3 months old because he was hard to wake up for feedings, drank very little milk, had gained less than a pound since birth, and had become increasingly weak. After the medical examination and tests failed to reveal any medical illness that could explain his feeding difficulties and poor weight gain, a psychiatric consultation was requested. Mark's mother, Mrs. Meyer, explained to the psychiatrist in tears that she had tried to tell the pediatricians that there was something wrong with Mark, that he just did not seem hungry and would fall asleep during feedings, that she had tried everything to get him to eat and that she could not understand why they could not find the problem. She proceeded to describe how she would lie awake at night, worrying that Mark would die, that she would get up to check on him and wake him up to be sure that he was alive.

Mark was the first child of his parents, after Mrs. Meyer had lost two previous pregnancies. Mrs. Meyer had been on bed rest for the last 4 weeks of the pregnancy because of high blood pressure and premature labor, but the delivery was uneventful. Mark was born full-term and weighed 6 pounds and 9 ounces. Mrs. Meyer tried to breast-feed, but because Mark had a poor suck and often fell asleep after suckling for only a few minutes, her pediatrician recommended that she transition him to bottle feedings. Initially, Mark seemed to do better with the bottle, but he would never take more than 3 or 4 ounces at a time and then would fall asleep. Mrs. Meyer stated that she became very worried about his poor feeding and would try to feed him every 1 or 2 hours. However, when she woke him up for feedings, he often would start to cry and continue crying for more than an hour without her being able to calm him. Because Mark took in so little formula during the day, Mrs. Meyer started to wake him up at night, first to check on him and then to feed him. The night feedings became more and more stressful, because Mark would cry on being awakened and sometimes it took Mrs. Meyer hours to calm him. Mr. Meyer had moved into the guest room because he could not sleep with all the crying throughout the night, and he could not function at his work the next day. Mrs. Meyer admitted that she felt exhausted and frightened for her baby, and that she had become very irritable in her interactions with her husband.

After Mrs. Meyer agreed, mother and baby were observed and video-taped during feeding from behind a one-way mirror. Mrs. Meyer brought in Mark sleeping in her arms. She tried to wake him up by holding his little body upright, but in spite of his head wobbling around because of his poor head control, Mark did not wake up. Mrs. Meyer started to pinch his feet, and suddenly he started to cry, which quickly escalated into screams. Mrs. Meyer looked frightened and started to walk the room with Mark crying at her shoulder. After 15 minutes of crying, the psychiatrist intervened and asked one of the nurses to take Mark back to the unit, while she stayed with the mother and tried to comfort her. The psychiatrist explained to Mrs. Meyer that she and Mark had gotten into a very stressful pattern of feedings, and that both of them were exhausted and needed a break. She recommended that the nurses take over the feedings for a while and that Mrs. Meyer should go home and sleep at home during the night. She set up an appointment to meet with both parents the next day to discuss further treatment recommendations.

The nurses reported that indeed, it was very hard to wake up Mark for feedings, and that he would transition from being unresponsive to screaming almost immediately. They proposed to feed him in a quiet room on the unit and to use some gentle infant massage to gradually stimulate him and wake him. They also put him on a feeding schedule with 3-hour intervals to allow him to resume a normal sleep pattern and to get hungry for feedings. Mark responded well to these changes, and within a few days, he became more alert during feedings and started to take 4 to 5 ounces at a time. In the meantime, the psychiatrist met with the parents and learned that Mrs. Meyer could not sleep at night, cried often during the day, and blamed herself for Mark's feeding problems. Mr. Meyer tried to comfort and reassure her that she had done her best, but Mrs. Meyer was just overwhelmed with guilt. The psychiatrist explained to the parents that Mark started out having difficulty regulating sleep and wakefulness, which affected his feeding, and that mother and baby had adopted a cycle of very stressful interactions. She offered to refer Mrs. Meyer for treatment of her depression and Mrs. Meyer accepted the referral.

In the meantime, the nurses taught Mrs. Meyer how to stimulate Mark with gentle massage to help him with the transition from sleep to wakefulness, and as Mrs. Meyer became more confident, she gradually took over the feedings in the hospital. In addition to the nurses' intervention, a physical therapist worked with Mark and taught Mrs. Meyer how to do exercises at home in order to strengthen Mark's muscle tone. Mark was weighed daily and started to show gradual weight gain. After 2 weeks of treatment in the hospital, Mark seemed stronger, his feedings were better regulated, and Mrs. Meyer felt confident enough in her ability to feed Mark that he could be discharged home.

Mark and his mother continued to visit the psychiatrist on a weekly basis for a few weeks and then biweekly for a few more months to videotape the feedings and to discuss Mark's behavior. Mrs. Meyer gradually recovered from her depression and became increasingly confident in her ability to read Mark's cues and to care for him. Mark showed a gradual improvement in his appetite, and by 6 months he was "back on the growth chart," meaning he had normalized his weight. He continued to require a significant amount of sleep and functioned well with a regular schedule of two naps during the day and an early bedtime. He was a sensitive boy who when upset cried intensely and required time to calm himself, but with his mother's understanding of this vulnerability, he improved, and was a delightful little boy at 6 months old.

Differential Diagnosis

Feeding Disorder of State Regulation should be a diagnosis of exclusion after organic conditions that can interfere with state regulation of the infant have been ruled out. As Roberts, Ostapchuk, and O'Brien (2004) point out, 5% of infants presenting with excessive crying were found to have underlying organic conditions. Most notably, gastroesophageal reflux needs to be considered in the differential diagnosis. As described in more detail in the chapter on Feeding Disorder Associated With a Concurrent Medical Condition, infants with "silent" gastroesophageal reflux may not vomit but cry excessively, become distressed during feedings, arch themselves, and refuse to continue feeding. If infants are observed to feed only small amounts and fall asleep during feedings, cardiac or respiratory conditions should be considered in the differential diagnosis. The additional diagnosis of Feeding Disorder of State Regulation should be considered if treatment of the organic problem, such as cardiac or pulmonary disease, cannot resolve the infant's difficulty in state regulation.

References

Canivet, C., Jakobsson, I., & Hagander, B. (2000). Infantile colic. Follow-up at four years of age: Still more "emotional." *Acta Paediatrica, 89*, 13–17.

Chatoor, I., & Ammaniti, M. (2007). A classification of feeding disorders of infancy and early childhood. In W. E. Narrow, M. B. First, P. Sirovatka, & D. A. Regier (Eds.), *Age and gender considerations in psychiatric diagnosis: A research agenda for DSM-V* (pp. 227–242). Arlington, VA: American Psychiatric Press.

Chatoor, I., Dickson, L., Schaefer, S., & Egan, J. (1985). A developmental classification of feeding disorders associated with failure-to-thrive: Diagnosis and treatment. In D. Drotar (Ed.), *New directions in failure to thrive: Research and clinical practice* (pp. 235–258). New York: Plenum.

Chatoor, I., Getson, P., Menvielle, E., O'Donnell, R., Rivera, Y., Brasseaux, C., & Mrazek, D. (1997). A feeding scale for research and clinical practice to assess mother-infant interactions in the first three years of life. *Infant Mental Health Journal, 18*, 76–91.

Lindberg, L., Bohlin, G., & Hagekull, B. (1991). Early feeding problems in a normal population. *The International Journal of Eating Disorders, 10*, 395–405.

McKenzie, S. (1991). Troublesome crying in infants: Effects of advice to reduce stimulation. *Archives of Disease in Childhood, 66*, 1416–1420.

Miller-Loncar, C., Bigsby, R., High, P., Wallach, M., & Lester, B. (2004). Infant colic and feeding difficulties. *Archives of Disease in Childhood, 89*, 908–912.

Narrow, W. E., First, M. B., Sirovatka, P., & Regier, D. A. (Eds.). (2007). *Age and gender considerations in psychiatric diagnosis: A research agenda for DSM-V.* Arlington, VA: American Psychiatric Press.

Roberts, D. M., Ostapchuk, M., & O'Brien, J. G. (2004). Infantile colic. *American Family Physician, 70*, 735–740.

Wessel, M. A., Cobb, J. C., Jackson, E. B., Harris, G. S., Jr., & Detwil, A. C. (1954). Paroxysmal fussing in infancy, sometimes called colic. *Pediatrics, 14*, 421–435.

ZERO TO THREE. (2005). *Diagnostic classification of mental health and developmental disorders of infancy and early childhood: Revised edition (DC:0–3R).* Washington, DC: Author.

Zwart, P., Vellema-Goud, M. G. A., & Brand, P. L. P. (2007). Characteristics of infants admitted to hospital for persistent colic, and comparison with healthy infants. *Acta Paediatrica, 96*, 401–405.

FEEDING DISORDER OF CAREGIVER–INFANT RECIPROCITY

Nosology

THIS FEEDING DISORDER is characterized by a lack of engagement between mother and infant, leading to inadequate food intake and growth failure of the infant. The symptoms of this feeding disorder are often referred to as *nonorganic failure to thrive* (NOFTT). Kim Oates (1984), in her excellent review of nonorganic failure to thrive, points out that the term should be used as a description rather than a diagnosis. However, it is often used as a diagnosis to characterize infants who show a decline from a previously established growth pattern and whose weight has fallen below the third percentile for age on standardized growth charts. Historically, Chapin (1915) was the first to report that growth failure and in some cases death were associated with emotional deprivation and lack of stimulation in children living in institutions. These findings were later confirmed by Spitz (1945) and Bakwin (1949). Coleman and Provence (1957) reported that the clinical syndrome of growth failure due to deprivation could also be observed in children living in their own homes. Most of the research on this syndrome of NOFTT due to maternal deprivation or neglect was published in the next 3 decades following their report.

Because several studies of infants with the diagnosis of NOFTT have demonstrated very high rates of insecure attachment, ranging from 50% to 90% of the infants studied (Gordon & Jameson, 1979; Valenzuela, 1990; Ward, Kessler, & Altman, 1993), the American Psychiatric Association (1980) defined this syndrome as "Reactive Attachment

Disorder of Infancy" associated with failure to thrive (FTT) in the *Diagnostic and Statistical Manual of Mental Disorders* (3rd ed.). The diagnostic criteria included lack of care that ordinarily leads to the development of affectional bonds to others, lack of developmentally appropriate signs of social responsivity, and weight loss or failure to gain appropriate amounts of weight. However, in the fourth edition of the *Diagnostic and Statistical Manual* (American Psychiatric Association, 1994), the same diagnosis was changed to encompass only problems in relatedness without growth failure, and the children diagnosed with growth failure and maternal deprivation as described earlier were captured under "Neglect of Child."

In my earlier publications, my colleagues and I described this feeding disorder as Feeding Disorder of Attachment (Chatoor, 1991; Chatoor, 2002; Chatoor, Dickson, Schaefer, & Egan, 1985; Chatoor, Getson, Menville, Brasseaux, & O'Donnell, 1997). However, because attachment is difficult to measure in the first year of life, on recommendation of the national Task Force for Research Diagnostic Criteria for Infants and Preschool Children (Scheeringa et al., 2003), I changed the label to *Feeding Disorder of Caregiver–Infant Reciprocity*. The diagnostic criteria for Feeding Disorder of Caregiver–Infant Reciprocity were further revised when I worked with the National Infant and Young Child Research Planning Work Group, which was supported by the American Psychiatric Association. These revised criteria for Feeding Disorder of Caregiver–Infant Reciprocity described below were included in *Diagnostic Classification of Mental Health and Developmental Disorders of Infancy and Early Childhood: Revised Edition* (*DC:0–3R*; ZERO TO THREE, 2005) and were described in Chatoor and Ammaniti's (2007) chapter in *Age and Gender Considerations in Psychiatric Diagnosis: A Research Agenda for DSM-V* (Narrow, First, Sirovatka, & Regier, 2007).

Diagnostic Criteria

A. This feeding disorder is usually observed in the first year of life, when the infant presents with some acute medical problem (commonly an infection) to the primary care physician or the emergency room, and the physician notices that the infant is malnourished.

B. The infant shows lack of developmentally appropriate signs of social reciprocity (e.g., visual engagement, smiling, or babbling) with the primary caregiver during feeding.

C. The infant shows significant growth deficiency.

D. The primary caregiver is often unaware or in denial of the feeding and growth problems of the infant.

E. The growth deficiency and lack of relatedness are not due solely to a physical disorder, or a pervasive developmental disorder.

Clinical Presentation

Having achieved some capacity for self-regulation, between 2 and 6 months of age, the adaptive infant is able to engage caretakers in an increasingly reciprocal relationship that is characterized by mutual eye contact, reciprocal vocalizations, and mutual physical closeness expressed through cuddling and holding. Because most of the infant's interactions with the caregiver occur around feeding, at this developmental stage, the regulation of food intake is closely linked to the infant's emotional engagement with the caregiver. If the infant and caregiver are not successfully engaged with each other, feeding and growth of the infant will suffer and impair the infant's emotional and cognitive development.

In my experience, this feeding disorder is often not detected until the infants become acutely ill and present to the pediatrician or to the emergency room. On examination, the pediatricians will find the infants to be malnourished and weak. When picked up, the infants often scissor their legs, stiffen their bodies, and assume a surrender posture to balance their heads, which seem to be too heavy for their small, malnourished, hypotonic bodies. Some infants are so weak and hypotonic that they resemble little rag dolls. Other authors have described them as having cold hands and feet; showing minimal smiling, decreased vocalizations, and apathetic and withdrawn behavior; and seeking indiscriminate affection when they are toddlers (Bullard, Glaser, Heagarty, & Pivchik, 1967; Leonard, Rhymes, & Soinit, 1966; Rosenn, Loeb, & Jura, 1980).

The mothers of these children are often difficult to engage, distrustful, and avoidant of any contact with professionals. When questioned about their infants' feeding and growth, they seem unaware or not willing to admit that there is a problem. However, I have encountered some mothers who revealed that they were overwhelmed by the care of other children, and that they were propping the bottles to feed the infant in order to save time while busy with their other children. In the literature, the mothers are often described as suffering from affective illness, alcohol abuse, drug abuse, character disorders, and poor health, and leading chaotic lifestyles (Evans, Reinhart, & Succop, 1972; Fischoff, Whitten, & Petit, 1971). They are also more likely to experience poverty and unemployment (Drotar & Malone, 1982) and have a history of abuse by their partners (Weston & Colloton, 1993). Clinicians and researchers have related the difficulty of these mothers to engage with their infants to their own deprivation in the past as well as their present relationship difficulties (Benoit, Zeanah, & Barton, 1989; Fraiberg, Anderson, & Shapiro, 1975).

Mother–infant interactions are characterized by a lack of mutual engagement and lack of pleasure in their relationship. The mothers frequently appear detached and not in tune with their babies. They often hold their infants loosely on their laps and appear depressed and in a different world, while the infants look away from their mothers and sometimes do not open their eyes while drinking from the bottle (Chatoor et al., 1997). Drotar, Eckerle, Satola, Pallotta, and Wyatt (1990) described how, during feedings, the mothers showed less socially adaptive behavior and had less positive affect, but most notably, demonstrated more arbitrary termination of feedings than a control group of mothers. These observations during feeding are most telling about the lack of engagement between mother and infant.

The following case illustrates some typical infant behaviors, maternal characteristics, and mother–infant interactions seen in Feeding Disorder of Caregiver–Infant Reciprocity.

Example: Jenny was 9 months old when she was brought to the emergency room by her parents, Mr. and Mrs. Brown, because of loose stools for the past 2 days. During the physical examination, Jenny hardly opened her eyes, which appeared sunken. Her hair looked thin and dirty, and her clothing was smelly and dirty. She could not hold up her head or sit up without support. Her little body was emaciated and dehydrated, but the rest of the physical examination was unremarkable. Jenny was admitted to the hospital and treated with intravenous saline solutions because of her dehydration and general weakness.

The parents reported that Jenny was their fourth child, the oldest only being 5 years old. Jenny was born full-term after an uneventful pregnancy and delivery, and she weighed 6 pounds and 4 ounces at birth. The family had just moved to the area a few months ago because Mr. Brown, who had been unemployed for more than a year, had been offered a job with a construction company that moved him and his family to this area. Soon after the parents had given this brief history and Jenny was admitted to the hospital, they were anxious to leave because they said their other children were sick with diarrhea as well.

Jenny's medical workup, including a stool culture, did not reveal any organic illness. However, the medical staff was concerned that Jenny was withdrawn and avoided eye contact, that her little body was limp like a rag doll, and that she lay in her bed with her eyes closed when alone. She would hardly cry if they had to draw blood, and when given the bottle, she had a weak suck and barely drank a few ounces of milk.

The parents did not visit Jenny for the next 4 days, and when the pediatrician and the nurses tried to call the parents, they found that the phone was disconnected. After they had been unable to reach the parents for 5 days, they notified Protective Services because of Jenny's poor hygiene on admission, her severe malnutrition, and the unavailability of the parents. They also requested a consultation by psychiatry to assess Jenny and her family.

With the help of Protective Services, the psychiatrist was able to set up an appointment with Mrs. Brown, to gain more information and to observe mother and infant during feeding and play. Mrs. Brown revealed that she was alone and did not know anybody in the area, and that she felt overwhelmed with the care of her four young children. She admitted to propping Jenny's bottles because she was so busy "chasing after the other children" and said that Jenny did not seem to mind. She admitted to drinking alcohol with Mr. Brown in the evening because that was the only way she could get through the evening and fall asleep. She revealed that her father used to drink and beat her when she was a child, and that she did not like that her husband "roughed up their children," but she could not express this to him.

Mother–infant interactions during feeding revealed a sad mother who stared into space while the infant lay listless in the mother's lap with her arms put back in a surrender position and her eyes closed while suckling from the bottle. During the play session, Mrs. Brown used the rattle to draw Jenny's attention, but Jenny was so weak that her head wobbled, she could not balance herself, and fell over. Mrs. Brown seemed unaware of Jenny's distress. She continued shaking the rattle while Jenny lay on the floor and whimpered softly.

Course of Feeding Disorder

Characteristically, infants like Jenny become engaging and gain weight when admitted to the hospital and put in the care of a nurturing nurse. However, several follow-up studies have demonstrated that these children are at risk not only for impaired growth but also for deficits in cognitive performance, behavioral organization, ego control, ego resiliency, and behavioral symptoms. Sturm and Drotar (1989) reported that of a sample of 3-year-old children who had been hospitalized for NOFTT as infants and received time-limited outreach intervention, nearly one third continued to demonstrate at least mild wasting. Shorter duration of NOFTT prior to the diagnosis and greater initial rate of weight gain following hospitalization predicted better weight for height at 36 months of age. A 5-year follow-up study of infants with NOFTT from Israel by Reif, Beler, Villa, and Spirer (1995) found that birth weight, maternal height, and social status were good predictors of catching-up capabilities of these infants in terms of weight and height. Children who caught up faster had better school performance and came from families of higher socioeconomic status.

Mackner, Starr, and Black (1997) proposed a model in which accumulation of risk factors is detrimental to cognitive development. In following a large sample of 3 to 30–month-old infants from clinics serving low-income families, they defined four groups based on neglect and FTT status: neglect and FTT, neglect only, FTT only, and no neglect or FTT. The cognitive performance of the group with neglect and FTT was significantly below that of the children in the neglect only, FTT only, and no neglect or FTT groups. Kerr, Black, and Krishnakumar (2000) reported later on the same cohort of children when they were 6 years old. They found that children with a history of both FTT and maltreatment had more behavioral problems and worse cognitive performance and school functioning than children with neither risk factor. Children with only one risk factor (either FTT or maltreatment) achieved intermediate scores.

In summary, infants with a Feeding Disorder of Caregiver–Infant Reciprocity are at high risk for ongoing problems in their physical, cognitive, and emotional development.

Etiology

As described above, the early literature referred to this feeding disorder as "maternal deprivation" (Fischoff et al., 1971; Patton & Gardner, 1963). It has been postulated that lack of emotional nurture and infrequent feedings lead to the growth failure and developmental delays of these infants. A prospective study of antecedents of NOFTT by Altemeier, O'Connor, Sherrod, and Vietze (1985) has shed some light on what may lead to the mothers' difficulty to engage with their infants. They found significant correlates with the mothers' aberrant nurture during their own childhood and conflicts between the parents of the infant. Bithoney and Newberger (1987) described social isolation of the mothers, few opportunities to escape caregiving, and fewer available extended family members as risk factors.

In summary, most studies indicate that the mothers have grown up in difficult circumstances without the nurture and security that would enable them to establish healthy relationships with others and to provide their infants with the nurture that they never received.

Treatment

Various treatment approaches have been proposed, ranging from home-based interventions to hospitalization in severe cases. In a controlled prospective study of infants with FTT by Black, Dubowitz, Hutcheson, Berenson-Howard, and Starr (1995), infants were randomly assigned to either a multidisciplinary feeding and nutrition clinic or to a home-based intervention by trained lay visitors. Although children in both types of intervention improved their growth pattern, the mothers in the home intervention created a more child-focused home environment for their children with FTT. In an intervention study that compared three treatment approaches (short-term assistance with social and economic problems, family-centered intervention, and parent-intervention), Sturm and Drotar (1989) found that none of the treatment methods was superior to the other in outcome.

Schmitt and Mauro (1989) considered an outpatient approach to be safe only in cases of mild neglect, if there is no evidence of deprivational behavior by the mother, if the infant is older than 12 months, if the parents have a support system, and if they have sought medical help for the infant for previous sickness. However, if the growth deficiency is more severe, if there is serious hygiene neglect, if the mother is abusing drugs or alcohol, or lives a chaotic lifestyle and appears overwhelmed with stress, or if the mother–infant interactions appear angry and uncaring, Schmitt and Mauro recommend immediate hospitalization.

During the hospitalization, several infant-directed interventions can occur while a more in-depth evaluation of the mother and the mother–infant relationship is taking place. It is critical to assign as few rotating nurses as possible to the infant and to have a warm and nurturing nurse take primary responsibility to engage the infant during feedings and play. Because many of the infants are severely hypotonic from lying in their cribs without being held or moved, it is very helpful to have a physical therapist work with the infant and teach the nurses and the mother how to move the infant to establish better muscle tone.

While the nutritional, emotional, and developmental rehabilitation of the infant takes place, the mother's ability to engage her infant and to participate in the treatment process needs to be assessed. Many of the mothers have experienced unsatisfactory relationships with their own caretakers when they were growing up, and consequently, they are distrustful and avoidant of professionals. It is important to identify any positive behavior the infant shows toward the mother to see whether the mother has any potential to engage in a mutually satisfying relationship with her infant. In addition, the mother's support system and her ability to become engaged with a therapist need to be explored prior to returning the infant to her care. The hospitalization of the infant provides a critical time to assess whether the infant needs to be placed in alternative care. In some situations of severe neglect and associated abuse, Protective Services need to be involved, which at times can be instrumental in mobilizing the family or in finding foster care.

Discharge from the hospital is a critical time when all services need to be in place in order to ensure follow-through of the treatment plan. The treatment plan should be individualized and may include home visits by a health care professional, day care for the infant, mother–infant psychotherapy, and family therapy for the parents. For some infants, day care in a nurturing environment will give the mother an opportunity to have some time for her own interests and needs and make the time with her infant more special and enjoyable. Visits by a home care nurse or a social worker, as first suggested by Fraiberg and colleagues (1975), to nurture the mother so she can nurture her infant, can break the mother out of her isolation and allow her to become more engaged with her child.

Interaction guidance, a treatment method developed by Susan McDonough (2004), is especially promising in helping these mothers and their babies. This treatment approach addresses family relationship problems by observing ongoing parent–infant interactive behavior and by providing guidance to the caregivers to gain a better understanding of their infant's and their own feelings, thoughts, and actions. By using videotape feedback and emphasizing family strengths, the infant's symptoms are reduced and the parents become empowered to develop a more mutually satisfying relationship with their infant.

The following case describes the diagnosis and treatment of an infant and his young mother who had experienced a deprived childhood, felt lonely and abandoned, and had very little to give to her infant.

Example: Carl was 8 months old when he was admitted to the hospital through the emergency room because of a respiratory tract infection and severe "failure to thrive." After he had recovered from the infection and a medical workup for his malnutrition was negative, a psychiatric consultation was requested. After repeated unsuccessful attempts, the psychiatrist finally reached the father, Mr. Long, and set up an appointment to obtain more history and to observe the mother and infant during feeding. Both parents attended the appointment. Mr. Long explained that he had difficulty obtaining time off from his construction job and that the mother, Miss Roberts, did not have any means of transportation to the hospital. The couple was not married because Mr. Long had not gotten his divorce from his first wife, but they lived together with Carl in one room in a house that they shared with nine other members of the father's extended family.

Miss Roberts had become pregnant with Carl during her last year of high school and had dropped out of school and moved in with Mr. Long. She described Carl as a quiet baby who slept a lot, but she denied any feeding problems. However, when Miss Roberts temporarily left the room, Mr.

Long turned to the psychiatrist and complained that Miss Roberts did not give enough attention to Carl, describing how she would talk on the phone or read a magazine while feeding the baby.

The observation of mother and infant during feeding revealed that the mother looked sad and preoccupied while she held her baby loosely on her lap. The infant lay in a "surrender position" with his arms raised beside his head, and he looked away while drinking from the bottle. However, when he looked at his mother, the mother looked away as if she could not tolerate eye contact with her infant.

Further evaluation of Miss Roberts revealed that she felt very lonely and depressed. She had been unable to finish high school because of the pregnancy with Carl. Her family had abandoned her for becoming involved with a married man. Her father was an alcoholic and had often beaten her when he was drunk. Her mother had never had time for her because she worked long hours as a cleaning lady. When she came home, she was tired and had to take care of Miss Roberts's four younger siblings. Miss Roberts described Mr. Long's family as hostile toward her. Mr. Long worked long hours and was rarely around. The telephone calls Miss Roberts made to her girlfriends from high school were the only relief in her unhappy life.

During the hospitalization, Carl gained weight, became more engaged, and rewarded his favorite nurse with frequent smiles. After the social worker had arranged for transportation for Miss Roberts, she regularly attended her appointments with the social worker and spent more time with Carl. In addition to nurturing Miss Roberts and trying to help her work on her situation with her own family and Mr. Long's family, the social worker also spent time with mother and infant during play. She would acknowledge how the baby was making progress, how he was trying to get his mother's attention, and how he had that special smile for his mother.

After 4 weeks in the hospital, Carl seemed stronger, and Miss Roberts seemed committed to continue working with the social worker. The hospital staff felt comfortable to discharge Carl. A nurse visited the home twice a week to check on mother and infant, and Miss Roberts and Carl attended weekly appointments at the hospital to see the social worker. After 6 months, the visiting nurse came less frequently, but Miss Roberts and Carl stayed in treatment with the social worker for another year when both seemed engaged and comfortable with each other.

Differential Diagnosis

This feeding disorder needs to be differentiated from organic conditions that lead to lack of weight gain and weakness of the infant. However, mother and infant usually show better mutual engagement, and the infant responds more readily to the examiner.

References

Altemeier, W. A., O'Connor, S. M., Sherrod, K. B., & Vietze, P. M. (1985). Prospective study of antecedents for nonorganic failure to thrive. *The Journal of Pediatrics, 106*(3), 360–365.

American Psychiatric Association. (1980). *Diagnostic and statistical manual of mental disorders* (3rd ed.). Washington, DC: Author.

American Psychiatric Association. (1994). *Diagnostic and statistical manual of mental disorders* (4th ed.). Washington, DC: Author.

Bakwin, H. (1949). Emotional deprivation in infants. *Journal of Pediatrics, 35*, 512–521.

Benoit, D., Zeanah, C. H., & Barton, M. L. (1989). Maternal attachment disturbances in failure to thrive. *Infant Mental Health Journal, 10*(3), 185–202.

Bithoney, W. G., & Newberger, E. H. (1987). Child and family attributes of failure-to-thrive. *Developmental and Behavioral Pediatrics, 8*(1), 32–36.

Black, M. M., Dubowitz, H., Hutcheson, J., Berenson-Howard, J., & Starr, R. H., Jr. (1995). A randomized clinical trial of home intervention for children with failure to thrive. *Pediatrics, 95*, 807–814.

Bullard, D. M., Glaser, H. H., Heagarty, M. C., & Pivchik, E. C. (1967). Failure to thrive in the neglected child. *American Journal of Orthopsychiatry, 37*, 680–690.

Chapin, H. D. (1915). Are institutions for infants necessary? *The Journal of the American Medical Association, 64*, 1–3.

Chatoor, I. (1991). Eating and nutritional disorders of infancy and early childhood. In J. Wiener (Ed.), *Textbook of child and adolescent psychiatry* (pp. 357–361). Washington, DC: American Psychiatric Press.

Chatoor, I. (2002). Feeding disorders in infants and toddlers: Diagnosis and treatment. *Child and Adolescent Psychiatric Clinics of North America, 11*, 163–183.

Chatoor, I., & Ammaniti, M. (2007). A classification of feeding disorders of infancy and early childhood. In W. E. Narrow, M. B. First, P. Sirovatka, & D. A. Regier (Eds.), *Age and gender considerations in psychiatric diagnosis: A research agenda for DSM-V* (pp. 227–242). Arlington, VA: American Psychiatric Press.

Chatoor, I., Dickson, L., Schaefer, S., & Egan, J. (1985). A developmental classification of feeding disorders associated with failure to thrive: Diagnosis and treatment. In D. Drotar (Ed.), *New directions in failure to thrive: Research and clinical practice* (pp. 235–238). New York: Plenum.

Chatoor, I., Getson, P., Menville, E., Brasseaux, C., & O'Donnell, R. (1997). A feeding scale for research and clinical practice to assess mother-infant interactions in the first three years of life. *Infant Mental Health Journal, 18*(1), 76–91.

Coleman, R. W., & Provence, S. (1957). Environmental retardation (hospitalism) in infants living in families. *Pediatrics, 19*, 285–292.

Drotar, D., Eckerle, D., Satola, J., Pallotta, J., & Wyatt, B. (1990). Maternal interactional behavior with nonorganic failure-to-thrive infants: A case comparison study. *Child Abuse & Neglect, 14*, 41–51.

Drotar, D., & Malone, C. A. (1982). Family-oriented intervention in fail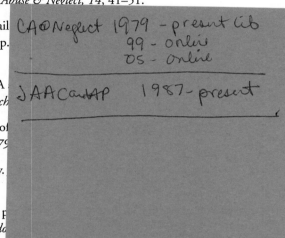 M. O. Robertson (Eds.), *Birth interaction and attachment* (6th ed., pp. Johnson & Johnson Pediatric Roundtable.

Evans, S. L, Reinhart, J. B., & Succop, R. A. (1972). Failure to thrive: A families. *Journal of the American Academy of Child and Adolescent Psych*

Fischoff, J., Whitten, C. F., & Petit, M. G. (1971). A psychiatric study of failure secondary to maternal deprivation. *The Journal of Pediatrics, 79*

Fraiberg, S., Anderson, E., & Shapiro, U. (1975). Ghosts in the nursery. *of Child and Adolescent Psychiatry, 14*, 387–421.

Gordon, A. H., & Jameson, J. C. (1979). Infant-mother attachment in p to thrive syndrome. *Journal of the American Academy of Child and Ado*

Kerr, M. A., Black, M. M., & Krishnakumar, A. (2000). Failure-to-thriv and development of 6-year-old children from low-income, urban fam *Child Abuse & Neglect, 24*, 587–598.

Leonard, M. F., Rhymes, J. P., & Soinit, A. J. (1966). Failure to thrive in infants: A family problem. *American Journal of Diseases of Children, 111*, 600–612.

Mackner, L. M., Starr, R. H., & Black, M. M. (1997). The cumulative effect of neglect and failure to thrive on cognitive functioning. *Child Abuse & Neglect, 21*, 691–700.

McDonough, S. C. (2004). Interaction guidance: Promoting and nurturing the caregiving relationship. In A. J. Sameroff, S. C. McDonough, & K. L. Rosennblum (Eds.), *Treating parent-infant relationship problems* (pp. 79–96). New York: Guilford.

Narrow, W. E., First, M. B., Sirovatka, P., & Regier, D. A. (Eds.). (2007). *Age and gender considerations in psychiatric diagnosis: A research agenda for DSM-V.* Arlington, VA: American Psychiatric Press.

Oates, R. K. (1984). Non-organic failure to thrive. *Australian Paediatric Journal, 20*, 95–100.

Patton, R. G., & Gardner, L. L. (1963). *Growth failure in maternal deprivation.* Springfield, IL: Charles C. Thomas.

Reif, S., Beler, B., Villa, Y., & Spirer, Z. (1995). Long-term follow-up and outcome of infants with non-organic failure to thrive. *Israel Journal of Medical Sciences, 31*, 483–489.

Rosenn, D. W., Loeb, L. S., & Jura, M. B. (1980). Differentiation of organic from non-organic failure to thrive syndrome in infancy. *Pediatrics, 66*, 698–704.

Scheeringa, M., Anders, T., Boris, N., Carter, A., Chatoor, I., Egger, H., et al. (2003). Research diagnostic criteria for infants and preschool children: The process and empirical support. *Journal of the American Academy of Child and Adolescent Psychiatry, 42*, 1504–1512.

Schmitt, B. D., & Mauro, R. D. (1989). Nonorganic failure to thrive: An outpatient approach. *Child Abuse & Neglect, 13*, 235–248.

Spitz, R. (1945). Hospitalism, an inquiry into the genesis of psychiatric conditions in early childhood. *The Psychoanalytic Study of the Child, 1*, 53–74.

Sturm, L., & Drotar, D. (1989). Prediction of weight for height following intervention in three-year-old children with early histories of nonorganic failure to thrive. *Child Abuse & Neglect, 13*, 19–28.

Valenzuela, M. (1990). Attachment in chronically underweight young children. *Child Development, 61*, 1984–1996.

Ward, M. J., Kessler, D. B., & Altman, S. C. (1993). Infant-mother attachment in children with failure to thrive. *Infant Mental Health Journal, 14*, 208–220.

Weston, J., & Colloton, M. (1993). A legacy of violence in nonorganic failure to thrive. *Child Abuse & Neglect, 17*, 709–714.

ZERO TO THREE. (2005). *Diagnostic classification of mental health and developmental disorders of infancy and early childhood: Revised edition (DC:0–3R)*. Washington, DC: Author.

CHAPTER 4

INFANTILE ANOREXIA

Nosology

IN 1983, my colleague James Egan and I first described a group of otherwise healthy toddlers who displayed severe food refusal and failure to thrive (FTT; growth deficiency) but who did not fit the description of what had been described in the literature as nonorganic failure to thrive (NOFTT; Chatoor & Egan, 1983). These toddlers showed no signs of maternal deprivation, which was thought to be the underlying cause of NOFTT. Quite to the contrary, the parents were concerned about their toddlers' poor food intake and had made multiple efforts to help their toddlers to eat more. Initially, we called this feeding disorder a separation disorder, because it seemed to develop during the developmental period of separation and individuation, when the toddlers were involved in intense struggles with their mothers over autonomy and control, especially during feeding but sometimes during play as well. Later, my colleagues and I (Chatoor, 1989; Chatoor, Egan, Getson, Menvielle, & O'Donnell, 1988) called this feeding disorder "Infantile Anorexia Nervosa" because of the similarities in the struggles for autonomy and control between Anorexia Nervosa and this feeding disorder. Consequently, my colleagues and I (Chatoor et al., 1992) changed the name to Infantile Anorexia to draw attention to the lack of appetite (anorexia) as the central symptom with the onset of this feeding disorder during infancy, and to differentiate it from Anorexia Nervosa, which is characterized by the fear of being or becoming overweight and has a later onset during childhood, adolescence, or adulthood.

The diagnostic criteria underwent some changes when I worked with the national Task Force for Research Diagnostic Criteria for Infants and Preschool Children (Scheeringa et al., 2003), which recommended that the caretaker–infant interactional criteria be omitted. The diagnostic criteria for Infantile Anorexia published in *Diagnostic Classification of Mental Health and Developmental Disorders of Infancy and Early Childhood: Revised Edition—DC:0–3R* (ZERO TO THREE, 2005) underwent some further minor modifications in the wording of some of the criteria. The diagnostic criteria were reviewed and further modified when I worked with the national Infant and Young Child Research Planning Work Group, which was supported by the American Psychiatric Association. These revised criteria for Infantile Anorexia and for five other feeding disorders presented in this book were described in Chatoor and Ammaniti's (2007) chapter in *Age and Gender Considerations in Psychiatric Diagnosis: A Research Agenda for DSM-V* (Narrow, First, Sirovatka, & Regier, 2007). The most recent diagnostic criteria for Infantile Anorexia are presented below.

Diagnostic Criteria

A. This feeding disorder is characterized by the infant's or toddler's refusal to eat adequate amounts of food for at least 1 month.

B. Onset of the food refusal often occurs during the transition to spoon and self-feeding, typically between 6 months and 3 years of age.

C. The infant or toddler rarely communicates hunger, lacks interest in food and eating, and would rather play, walk around, or talk than eat.

D. The infant or toddler shows significant growth deficiency (acute and/or chronic malnutrition according to Waterlow et al., 1977[1] or the child's weight deviates across two major percentiles in a 2–6-month period).

---

[1]Acute malnutrition, according to the Waterlow criteria (Waterlow et al., 2007), reflects current or "acute" nutritional status. The reference "normal" is the 50th percentile weight for the child's height. The child's current weight divided by this number gives the percentage of ideal body weight. Mild, moderate, and severe acute malnutrition corresponds with 80% to 89%, 70% to 79%, and less than 70% of ideal body weight, respectively.

Chronic malnutrition, according to the Waterlow criteria, defines stunting of linear growth. The child's actual height is divided by the height that corresponds to the 50th percentile of the growth chart of the National Center for Health Statistics for the age of the child. This number results in the child's percentage of "ideal height." Mild, moderate, and severe chronic malnutrition corresponds to 90% to 95%, 85% to 89%, and less than 85% of ideal height, respectively.

Additional parameters of faltering growth are reflected in the child's weight deviating across two major percentiles in a 2- to 6-month period. This measure is particularly helpful for children who start out tall, grow at the 50th or more percentile for weight and height, and then show a downward bent in their growth pattern.

E. The food refusal did not follow a traumatic event to the oropharynx or gastrointestinal tract.

F. The food refusal is not due to an underlying medical illness.

Clinical Presentation

Children with this feeding disorder are usually referred for a psychiatric evaluation because of food refusal and growth failure. When reviewing their feeding history, some mothers report that even during the first few months of life, these infants were easily distracted by external stimuli. If somebody entered the room, if the telephone rang, or even if the mother changed position, these infants would stop feeding, look around, and not want to resume feeding again. However, most parents describe that the onset of the feeding difficulties occurs during the transition to spoon- and self-feeding, between 9 and 18 months of age. The infants take only a few bites of food and then refuse to open their mouth for feeding. They throw food and feeding utensils, and frequently try to climb out of the high chair and run around. Most parents report that these children are active, playful, curious, and engaging, but hardly show any signals of hunger and are not interested in eating. Parents often describe that these children can go for hours or all day long and never signal that they are hungry and want to eat.

Often, the parents become increasingly worried about their infant's poor food intake and slow growth, and they try to encourage the child to eat by coaxing, distracting with toys and television, reading stories, offering different foods, feeding while the child is running around and playing, or feeding at night. Some parents get so desperate that they resort to threatening and even force-feeding. Sometimes distractions or offering different foods helps temporarily, but with the passage of time, the toddlers get bored with the toys and the parents have to come up with ever-new distractions. Some parents have reported that they were feeding their toddlers in the bathtub with water toys to keep them from running around. Others admitted that one parent was opening and closing umbrellas or jingling bells while the other parent slipped food into the toddler's mouth. While the parents resort to distractions and some of these desperate measures, the toddlers' eating becomes completely regulated externally through the interactions with their parents. This becomes an increasing burden for the parents, who end up feeling frustrated and helpless, because despite all of their efforts, the child's food intake remains inadequate for normal growth.

Initially the infants fail to gain adequate weight. After several weeks or months of poor food intake, their linear growth slows down and they develop chronic malnutrition, which is characterized by stunting of their height. Interestingly, in most cases, their heads continue to grow at a normal rate, and their cognitive development is age-appropriate, and sometimes even superior. As the children grow older, their bodies appear proportionate, small and thin, whereas their heads have the appropriate size for their age. A 4-year-old child may look like a toddler of 2 years, or a 9-year-old might be mistaken for a first grader. However, there are some children who continue to grow at a normal rate but become extremely thin because of their poor food intake.

The following example illustrates the development of food refusal and growth deficiency in a toddler with Infantile Anorexia:

Example: Susan was 17 months old when she was referred by her pediatrician to the Multidisciplinary Feeding Disorders Team for an evaluation because of food refusal and faltering of her growth. Susan's weight had dropped from the 40th percentile at 9 months of age to the 5th percentile, and her height had dropped from the 50th percentile to the 20th percentile. However, her head circumference remained at the 50th percentile. In spite of her faltering growth, Susan was an active and engaging toddler. She had a vocabulary of more than 10 words, and she enjoyed playing and looking at her baby books.

Susan's parents, Mr. and Mrs. Ward, reported that she was a full-term baby and weighed 7 pounds and 8 ounces at birth. She had no medical problems, fed well from the breast without any difficulties, and grew along the 40th percentile for weight and the 50th percentile for height and head circumference until about 9 months old. However, Mrs. Ward reported that even at 2 months, Susan stopped feeding and looked around if somebody entered the room or if the phone rang. Consequently, Susan's mother moved her breast-feedings to the bedroom and used a diaper to shield Susan's eyes to keep her from being distracted, and generally the feedings went well.

At age 6 months, Mrs. Ward introduced Susan to cereal and baby food, which she accepted without difficulties. However, her mother noticed that after a few spoonfuls, Susan started to become restless, refused to open her mouth, and tried to grab the spoon from her mother. Mrs. Ward started to offer Susan various toys that seemed to keep her busy for a while and allowed her to be fed from the spoon while she played. However, starting at about 9 months old, Susan became increasingly resistant to opening her mouth, and her mother had to work harder and harder to keep Susan distracted while feeding her. Susan's mother resorted to using television, specifically a special videotape, which seemed to mesmerize Susan. However, the moment Susan became aware of being fed, she grabbed the spoon and threw it. At 11 months of age, Susan learned to walk and resisted being placed in the high chair. Even if Mrs. Ward managed to get Susan in the high chair, she would sit only for a short while and then start throwing food and feeding utensils, and struggle to get out of the high chair. Consequently, Mrs. Ward started to feed Susan "on the run." She would keep food out, and periodically she would offer Susan some food or follow Susan with the spoon. Susan was very playful and active but ate very little, and her major source of nutrition remained her breast-feeding, which she demanded up to eight times a day, plus two to three breast-feedings at night.

When the pediatrician saw Susan for her 12-month checkup, Susan had gained only a few ounces since she was 9 months old, although her height and head circumference continued to be at the 50th percentile. The pediatrician expressed concern and recommended that Mrs. Ward cut down on the breast-feeding in order to get Susan to eat more solid food. Following this visit, the mother became increasingly anxious, because Susan would throw temper tantrums if her mother withheld the breast, and she continued to eat very little solid food. The breast-feedings were usually rather short, just a few minutes, and the mother felt that Susan seemed to need the breast-feedings for comfort, and to be close to her mother, rather than because she was hungry. Feeding times became increasingly difficult, with struggles to get Susan in the high chair and to get any food into her. However, in spite of her poor eating, Susan seemed to be an active and happy toddler, as long as she did not have to eat. She enjoyed playing with her parents and demanded almost constant attention. Mrs. Ward was a professional and had planned to go back to work when Susan was 1 year old, but because of Susan's feeding difficulties and her clinging to her mother, Mrs. Ward decided to continue staying home to take care of Susan. She feared that nobody else could put up with Susan's difficult behavior around feeding, and she felt unable to withhold breast-feedings out of fear that Susan would starve and die. Mrs. Ward felt helpless and had convinced herself that she must have done something very wrong as a mother, that she had failed her child.

Some toddlers like Susan engage in increasingly intense food refusal, and sometimes pediatricians become so concerned about the toddlers' poor growth that they insert nasogastric feeding tubes, which are often pulled out by the toddlers. Intense struggles ensue when the tubes have to be reinserted by the parents. These struggles can lead to the child having a Posttraumatic Feeding Disorder (see chapter 6). In addition, the tube feedings further interfere with the child's awareness of hunger and make it even more difficult to help the child recognize hunger feelings. This makes it very difficult to remove the feeding tube when the child's weight has been restored.

The following case illustrates the effect of tube feeding on a toddler with Infantile Anorexia and the distress experienced by her parents:

Example: Anna was first seen for a diagnostic evaluation when she was 22 months old because of severe resistance to feeding and food refusal. She had a history of lack of interest in feeding and food refusal starting around 10 months of age. By 15 months, she had "fallen off the growth chart," and the pediatrician referred Anna to a behavioral feeding program, where she was rewarded for food acceptance by being given a toy for a short period of time and punished for food refusal by withholding of the toy. This feeding program resulted in increased crying of the child during feedings and in further growth deceleration. When Anna was 20 months old, the pediatrician became so concerned about her poor growth that she instituted nasogastric tube feedings. The parents were trained to insert the feeding catheter through the nose into Anna's stomach, and they were instructed to give Anna three bolus feedings during the day and continuous tube feedings during the night.

Anna would scream and fight her parents so intensely during this procedure that one parent had to wrap her in a blanket and hold her, while the other parent inserted the feeding tube and taped the tube to Anna's cheek. Sometimes, when Anna was only briefly unobserved, she would pull out the feeding tube, and the parents had to go through the whole procedure all over again. Although the tube feedings resulted in good weight gain, Anna and her parents were deeply traumatized by the procedure. Anna stopped accepting any food by mouth and would cry when she saw feeding utensils and food, or when she was positioned for feedings or for the insertion of the feeding tube. The father reported that he would experience palpitations on his drive home in anticipation of the insertion of the feeding tube. The mother felt totally exhausted from watching over her daughter and worrying about her daughter's weight.

Course and Natural History

A longitudinal research study by Dahl and colleagues in Sweden (Dahl, 1987; Dahl, Rydell, & Sundelin, 1994) demonstrated that food refusal associated with growth failure at 10 months of age often persists over time and that 70% of those children continued to have eating problems at home and at school when 7 years old. In addition, the prospective study by Marchi and Cohen (1990) found that there was a significant correlation between picky eating (defined as "does not eat enough," "is often or very often choosy about food," "usually eats slowly," and "is usually not interested in food") during the early years and Anorexia Nervosa during adolescence. The same cohort of approximately 800 children was followed again over a 17-year interval from early childhood to adulthood by Kotler, Cohen, Davies, Pine, and Walsh (2001). These authors identified eating conflicts, struggles with food, and unpleasant meals in early childhood as risk factors for the later development of eating disorders. Yet again, although some of these criteria of "picky eating" fit Infantile Anorexia, the findings need to be viewed with caution and cannot be fully translated into the outcome for Infantile Anorexia.

A longitudinal study of Infantile Anorexia by Lucarelli, Cimino, Petrocchi, and Ammaniti (2007) in Rome followed children who were initially diagnosed when they were between 6 months and 3 years old. The children were reexamined when they were 4–6 years old and again when 7–8 years old. Although there was improvement in their nutritional status, at 4–6 years of age, 46% continued to show mild, 22% moderate, and 13% severe degrees of malnutrition, and at 7–8 years of age, 58% showed mild and 21% moderate malnutrition. Only 21% of the children had normalized their weight. Most of the children continued to show ongoing eating problems, eating excessively slowly and avoiding new foods. In addition, when compared with a control group, they presented with more separation anxiety, school phobia, sleep disturbances, somatic complaints, and oppositional behaviors.

In my clinical experience with school-age children whose eating problems had started when they were toddlers but had not received any intervention, the conflict over eating between parents and toddlers continued into childhood. My clinical observation revealed that even when the children grow older, they do not seem to notice when they are hungry and would rather play than eat. They are often social children who like the company of friends, and they are curious children who enjoy learning and usually do well in school. Some of them state that "eating is boring" and that "they do not have any time to eat at school because during lunch is the only time they get to talk to their friends." Most boys and some of the girls are very unhappy about their small size, whereas some other girls seem confused about their body and may worry that their stomach is too big or their legs are becoming fat, not unlike adolescent girls with Anorexia Nervosa.

As I mentioned earlier, when children with Infantile Anorexia grow older, most of them grow very slowly, and their bodies appear proportionate, but short and thin, whereas their heads have the appropriate size for their age. Some children grow at a normal rate but become very thin. However, my clinical experience indicates that with improved food intake, the children maintain the capacity to reach full growth potential until the end of puberty, when their growth lines close.

The following case illustrates the possibility for catch-up growth, once the child eats more:

Example: John was 13½ years old when he was referred by his pediatrician for a psychiatric evaluation because of poor growth and severe conflicts with his mother over eating. John had the height and the bone age of a 9-year-old and had been excluded from all team sports at school because of his small stature. John had been seen by three different endocrinologists over the past several years, but they all found that he had normal growth hormone production and concluded that his growth deficiency was secondary to his poor food intake.

John's mother, Mrs. Hunter, recalled that she had struggled with him over eating since he was 8 months old and refused to be fed by her. She expressed deep frustration that he would bring home his lunches from school and say that he did not have time to eat at school. At home, he would rather play than eat and would argue when he was called to the table at mealtime. John explained that he just did not feel hungry and did not want to be bothered by his mother about eating. However, he was very distressed because of the teasing about his small size by his peers and his exclusion from team sports by the coaches. He was an excellent student, and he enjoyed the respect of his peers and his teachers because of his intellect and wit.

John was engaged in treatment and worked on reading his hunger and satiety cues to improve his caloric intake. He learned to disengage from the battles over food with his mother and was pleased with his accelerated growth once he started to eat more. When John was 19 years old and in college, his mother reported to me that John was doing well and had grown to be the tallest in the family.

General Demographic Characteristics

It is of interest that the studies by Ammaniti, Cimino, Lucarelli, Speranza, and Vismara (2004) in Rome and by Chatoor and colleagues (Chatoor, Ganiban, Hirsch, Borman-Spurrell, & Mrazek, 2000; Chatoor, Hirsch, Ganiban, Persinger, & Hamburger, 1998) in Washington, DC, showed that Infantile Anorexia occurs with the same frequency in boys and girls, in contrast to Anorexia Nervosa, which is seen predominantly in females. In addition, both sites found that the referred children came predominantly from the middle- and upper-middle-class, which has been reported for Anorexia Nervosa as well. This may be a consequence of the referral pattern, because both sites operate specialty clinics, and lower-class families may have more difficulty accessing specialty services for their children. It may also be that lower- class families have so many other struggles for survival that they do not have the energy to worry about the child's food intake.

Child Characteristics

Temperament

A few studies have found that toddlers with Infantile Anorexia are rated by their parents as more negative, irregular, dependent, unstoppable, and difficult (Chatoor et al., 2000), and they exhibit more anxiety/depression, somatic complaints, and aggressive behaviors than healthy control children (Ammaniti, Ambruzzi, Lucarelli, Cimino, & D'Olimpio, 2004). As indicated by these studies, many of the toddlers with Infantile Anorexia demonstrate a difficult temperament characterized by irregular feeding and sleeping patterns, unstoppable and willful behavior, intense temper tantrums, increased dependency on their mothers, and severe separation anxiety. Although not all of the toddlers with Infantile Anorexia show all of these temperament characteristics, the study by Chatoor et al. (2000) showed a significant correlation between difficult toddler temperament characteristics and the intensity of mother–toddler conflict during feeding. In addition, both mother–toddler conflict during feeding and difficult toddler temperament characteristics showed a strong correlation with the toddlers' weight. The more difficult toddlers demonstrated more intense conflict with their mothers during feeding and presented with lower weights. Although this was a cross-sectional study, and one cannot determine the direction of the correlation, clinical case histories support the assumption that difficult toddler characteristics lead to a more severe expression of Infantile Anorexia.

Physiological Arousal

A pilot study by Chatoor, Ganiban, Surles, and Doussard-Roosevelt (2004) found increased physiological arousal and decreased ability to modulate physiological reactivity in toddlers with Infantile Anorexia compared with a control group of healthy eaters. This study was initiated because of the clinical observation that toddlers with Infantile Anorexia appear to go for long periods of time without signaling that they experience hunger, and the parents usually need to urge the children to eat because they feel that the children are not aware of hunger feelings. At the same time, these toddlers are very "busy" children who are constantly "on the go." They have difficulty interrupting their play in order to eat, and they seem to seek cognitive stimulation and find distractions when they are seated in the high chair, instead of relaxing and eating. Many of the children also have difficulty turning off the stimulation and relaxing when they need to go to sleep. These toddlers seem to be in a physiological "overdrive" that facilitates cognitive and physical activity, and they have difficulty down-regulating this physiological arousal, which is necessary for eating, sleeping, and growth.

This study raises the question of whether the difficulty of recognizing hunger, which characterizes children with Infantile Anorexia, may be related to a different physiological arousal pattern, that is, that these children do not feel hunger because of their heightened physiological arousal. This study should be replicated with larger numbers of children to further explore this important question.

Toddlers' Attachment Security

Additional studies have found that toddlers with Infantile Anorexia exhibited a higher rate of insecure attachment relationships than healthy eaters (Ammaniti, Cimino, et al., 2004; Chatoor, Ganiban, et al., 1998) although the majority of anorexic toddlers (60%) showed secure attachment patterns. However, the significant correlation between the severity of malnutrition and the degree of attachment insecurity indicated that an insecure toddler–mother relationship is associated with a more severe expression of Infantile Anorexia (Chatoor, Ganiban, et al.).

Toddlers' Cognitive Development

A study by Chatoor, Surles, et al. (2004) demonstrated that, on average, toddlers with Infantile Anorexia performed within the normal range of cognitive development. However, this study revealed that the Mental Developmental Index (MDI) scores of the healthy eaters were significantly higher than those of the Infantile Anorexia group. Within the Infantile Anorexia group, correlations between MDI scores and the toddlers' percentage ideal body weight did not reach statistical significance, whereas across all groups, the toddlers' MDI scores showed a significant correlation with the quality of mother–child interactions, the educational level of the mother, and the socioeconomic status of the family. The more conflict that mother and child experienced during feeding and play, the lower was the MDI of the child. The higher the mother's education and the socioeconomic level of the family, the better the child performed during the developmental testing.

This study is of major clinical significance because pediatricians are often most concerned about the child's "failure to thrive," fearing that the growth deficiency will lead to intellectual impairment when the child grows older. This study demonstrated that it is not the child's weight but the interactions between mother and child during feeding and play that threaten the child's development. Consequently, it is very important to listen to the parents' distress about the child's food refusal and not focus exclusively on the child's weight.

Parent Characteristics

When dealing with infants and young children, understanding the contributions of parental psychopathology and poor parenting skills to the distress and impairment of the child is of utmost importance. However, no prospective longitudinal studies that address this connection are available. Cross-sectional studies by Chatoor et al. (2000) and by Ammaniti, Cimino, et al. (2004) shed some light on specific characteristics of mothers that may be associated with their children's feeding disorder.

Given that parenting behavior is often transmitted from one generation to the next, the study by Chatoor and colleagues (2000) examined the attachment patterns of mothers to their own parents in (a) mothers of toddlers with Infantile Anorexia, (b) mothers of toddlers who were considered "picky eaters," and (c) mothers of healthy eaters. The authors found that more mothers of toddlers with Infantile Anorexia demonstrated insecure attachment patterns to their own parents than did mothers of picky eaters and mothers of healthy control children. In addition, insecure attachment in the mother was related to the intensity of conflict between mother and child during feeding. This indicated that insecure mothers are more likely to engage in conflict, and they struggle more intensely with their anorexic toddlers. However, it is important to remember that not all mothers of anorexic toddlers demonstrate insecure attachment patterns and are still drawn into food battles with their anorexic toddlers.

The study by Ammaniti, Cimino, et al. (2004) focused more on parental psychopathology and found more dysfunctional eating attitudes, anxiety, depression, and hostility in mothers of anorexic children than in mothers of healthy control children. Again, this was a cross-sectional study, and not all mothers of the anorexic children demonstrated psychopathology.

Caretaker–Toddler Interactions

Further studies have revealed that in Infantile Anorexia, mother–toddler interactional patterns are characterized by less dyadic reciprocity, high dyadic conflict, struggle for control, and increased talk and distractions during feedings (Chatoor et al., 1988; Chatoor, Ganiban, Harrison, & Hirsch, 2001; Chatoor, Getson, et al., 1997; Chatoor, Hirsch, et al., 1998; Lucarelli, Ambruzzi, Cimino, D'Olimpio, & Finistrella, 2003). These observations, which were replicated in several studies not only in our center but also by another team in Rome, are very important in understanding this feeding disorder. Therefore, observation of the primary caretaker and the toddler during feeding should be an essential part of the assessment. The observations revealed the intensity of the toddler's food refusal and the way the parent copes with it. As mentioned earlier, often the toddler is easily distracted, refuses to open his mouth, throws food and feeding utensils, struggles to get out of the high chair, and runs around the room, while the parent tries to get some food into the toddler's mouth by playing games, distracting him, running after the toddler with the spoon, or becoming forceful, holding the toddler down, and pushing food into his mouth.

The following case illustrates how the conflict between mother and toddler can escalate and lead to force-feeding:

Example: Albert was 15 months old when he was referred by his pediatrician because of food refusal and faltering growth. His mother, Mrs. Harris, reported that she started to get worried about Albert's eating when he was 8 months old. He was very precocious in his motor development and was already walking along the furniture at that time. He just wanted to move around and protested being put in the high chair. When Mrs. Harris got him settled in the high chair, he refused to open his mouth, grabbed the spoon from her, and threw it away. Albert's mother gave up on the high chair and tried to feed him while he was walking around and playing with his toys. As he became more active, it became increasingly difficult to get any amount of food into him, and his major caloric intake came from his bottle feedings. The bottle feedings also became less frequent during the day, and Albert would wake up two to three times at night and demand the bottle. At the time of the assessment, Mrs. Harris was exhausted and felt trapped by Albert's feeding pattern.

The observation of feeding revealed intense conflict between mother and child. Mrs. Harris managed to seat Albert in the high chair, and while he started reaching for the food and feeding utensils on the tray, she moved the tray further away and out of his reach. She attempted to feed him by spoon, but he batted the spoon away. She then gave him a french fry, which he also threw away, crying and reaching for the tray with the food that his mother had put out of his reach. While asking him, "What do you want?" Mrs. Harris offered him the spoon and some more french fries, but

Albert cried louder and threw everything away, while reaching for the food tray. Finally, Mrs. Harris held him down and pushed a french fry into his mouth. Albert screamed loudly and spit out every little piece of the french fry that his mother had put in his mouth. He was so distressed that he could not calm himself for the next 20 minutes.

Etiology

During my many years of clinical practice, I have seen 12 twin pairs with at least one child having Infantile Anorexia. Only one pair were identical twins, whereas the others were fraternal twins. It is interesting to note that both identical twins presented with Infantile Anorexia, whereas only in one pair of fraternal twins both children had symptoms of Infantile Anorexia, one child meeting full criteria and the other child having subthreshold symptoms. In the remaining 10 fraternal twin pairs, only one child had symptoms of Infantile Anorexia, whereas the other child was a good eater. These findings speak to a strong genetic component in the development of this feeding disorder.

In addition, often one or the other parent or a close relative of the child with Infantile Anorexia is found to have had similar feeding difficulties as a child, although not of the same severity as the presenting child. The parent who had similar feeding issues as a child often admits that when busy he or she forgets to eat, and that when having stressful life experiences he or she cannot eat. Together with the study findings of heightened physiological arousal in toddlers with Infantile Anorexia, I hypothesize that the heightened physiological arousal and difficulty in down-regulating when cognitively or emotionally stimulated present a biological vulnerability in infants who develop Infantile Anorexia. However, this hypothesis needs to be tested in further research.

The studies described above revealed specific temperament characteristics of the child and certain vulnerabilities of the parent to be associated with Infantile Anorexia, and both child and parent characteristics were significantly correlated to the strained parent–child relationship during feeding. As all of these studies were cross-sectional, they do not allow any firm conclusions about the causality of this feeding disorder. However, the developmental histories of these children reveal that from early infancy, these children display little interest in feeding and eat only small amounts, triggering parental anxiety and setting the stage for the ensuing parent–child struggles during feeding. Consequently, I have developed *a transactional model for Infantile Anorexia*. According to this model, infants with a poor hunger drive and refusal to eat elicit anxiety especially in the mothers who try to compensate for their infants' poor food intake by engaging in "noncontingent," inappropriate behaviors. These behaviors may range from distracting the toddler with toys or television while feeding to forcing food into the toddler's mouth. These parental behaviors further interfere with the toddler's awareness of hunger and lead to increasingly conflictual interactions between mother and child, who are both struggling for control. As a result of these struggles, the child does not learn to regulate eating internally. Eating becomes completely dependent on the interactions of the child with the caretakers.

This transactional model has served as a basis for an intervention described by Chatoor, Hirsch, and Persinger (1997) as facilitating internal regulation of eating in toddlers with Infantile Anorexia. I will describe this treatment model in the following section.

Treatment

The goal of the treatment is to facilitate the toddler's internal regulation of eating according to hunger and fullness. The treatment is based on the transactional model for Infantile Anorexia described above.

This model has three components that are addressed in the treatment:

1. The parents are helped to understand the toddler's special temperament, his high level of arousal and difficulty down-regulating, his difficulty in the perception of physiological hunger and satiety, and his curiosity and "intense hunger for stimulation and parental attention."

2. The parents' own eating history is explored to help the parents relate to the toddler's difficulty in the perception of hunger, and their experience with their own parents when growing up is reviewed to better understand the difficulties the parents may experience in setting limits to the toddler's provocative behaviors that interfere with feeding.

3. The parents are provided a set of specific feeding guidelines on how to structure mealtimes, and they are given instructions how to use time-out to help the toddler learn self-calming when he cannot have his way.

Understanding the Toddler's Special Temperament

The therapist combines the parents' description of their child with her own observations and highlights certain behaviors that are characteristic of the toddler. She may highlight how curious the toddler is, that his attention seemed to be so strongly focused on the pictures on the wall or his image in the mirror that he seemed to forget about the food in front of him. She may point out that it seemed more important for the toddler to engage his mother by asking her for all the different foods he could see, instead of putting the food in front of him in his mouth.

The therapist will share her observations of the toddler's difficulty staying in the high chair and relate it to his overall difficulty to settle and relax while eating. Then she will explain the finding of our study that toddlers with Infantile Anorexia seem to have a higher level of physiological arousal and that they have difficulty down-regulating their arousal when they need to eat or go to sleep. She will explain that this different physiological arousal pattern may be related to the toddler's difficulty experiencing hunger for food and explain his intense hunger for stimulation and for his parents' attention. She will sum it up by saying that "their toddler seems to have a big appetite for everything in the world except food."

Exploring the Parents' Eating Patterns

After these explanations, the therapist may inquire about the parents' regulation of eating and sleep. She may find that one or the other parent experienced similar difficulties in the regulation of eating and sleep. The parent may reveal that he or she forgets to eat when busy and may go for many hours until recognizing that he or she has not eaten anything for the day. Some parents may report that they see themselves running in "high drive," that they skip meals because they are too busy, and that they have difficulty relaxing or going to sleep until they are exhausted. These exchanges should help the parents to better understand their child and to see the child's behavior in a different light. At the end, the therapist will emphasize that the goal of the treatment will be for the parents to help their child to learn to recognize hunger and fullness and to eat accordingly.

Understanding the Parents' Background

This part of the interview focuses on building a strong therapeutic alliance with the parents to help them overcome the difficulties they may have in setting appropriate limits to their toddler's behaviors that interfere with feeding. The therapist wants to gain a better understanding of the parents' upbringing and other significant experiences, and the effect these experiences may have had on the parenting of their child. After encouraging the parents to look at themselves as children of their own parents, the therapist introduces their role as parents and asks them whether certain aspects of parenthood have been particularly difficult for them. The parents may admit how worried and helpless they feel when the child throws food and feeding utensils or climbs out of the high chair. This feeling of helplessness can often be linked to harsh discipline on the part of their own parents or to a fear of not being nurturing to their child because they experienced their own parents as unavailable and noncaring. Frequently, the parents want to be the parents they never had, and this wish tends to push them to the other extreme of what they experienced with their own parents.

On the other hand, for those parents who report secure relationships with their own parents, the therapist reinforces these positive experiences and explores other reasons that may make parenting so difficult with this child. Other common factors that may burden parents include the fear that the infant may starve to death because of their experience of previous losses, such as infertility problems, miscarriages, or the death of a close relative. The therapist must be flexible and try to understand why the parents are so anxious and overwhelmed by guilt that they have been ineffective in dealing with their child.

The Feeding Guidelines

After this groundwork has been laid, the parents are provided with specific guidelines on how to structure mealtimes and how to help their child learn internal regulation of eating. The parents are encouraged to work together on the implementation of the feeding guidelines because the young child's eating is easily modeled after the parents' eating. Children with Infantile Anorexia are generally very perceptive and use one parent against the other, if the parents are not in agreement with each other on how to handle mealtimes.

In the introduction to the specific guidelines, the therapist explains the principle of internal versus external regulation. The therapist points out that the child has learned to eat in response to external events and experiences with his parents, and instead he needs to learn to respond to his internal signals of hunger and fullness.

1. **To create stronger hunger cues, the parents are encouraged to feed the toddler at regular 3–4-hour intervals and not to offer any snack, milk, or juice in between. If the toddler is thirsty, he should be offered water.**

Toddlers with Infantile Anorexia can feel satisfied when they drink a few sips of juice, drink an ounce or two of milk, or eat a small amount of snack food, and they may not want to eat any more when mealtime approaches. Consequently, the implementation of regular mealtimes and no feeding in between is critical for toddlers to develop an awareness of hunger. However, it is often very difficult for parents to implement this first guideline because it requires lifestyle changes for the family to get on a regular meal schedule, and it is hard for parents to deny the toddler food outside of mealtimes because of their constant worry that the toddler is not eating enough. Therefore, it is helpful to go over the daily meal schedule for the family and tell the parents how to structure mealtimes so that they are sharing their meals with the child. Because many fathers tend to come home later and are often not part of the dinner, it is extremely important to set a meal schedule that includes the father. For many families this goes as follows: breakfast at around 8:00 a.m., lunch at noon, an afternoon snack (in the high chair) at 3:00 or 3:30, and dinner at 6:30. This schedule sets the stage for family dinners and supports the important role of the father during mealtimes. In addition, the parents need to be forewarned that initially the toddler may not eat much at mealtime but then demand the bottle or want to breast-feed an hour later. The parents need to be helped to tell the child that he has to wait until the next meal and to distract him; if the child throws a temper tantrum, the parents need to put him in time-out (which is described in detail on page 46) to calm himself. Children learn very quickly when the rules change and usually adapt to the new schedule as long as the parents are consistent with limit setting.

2. **The parents are to offer the toddler very small portions of food and allow her to ask for second, third, and fourth helpings to keep her engaged in the eating process and to prevent her from becoming bored or overwhelmed by the large amount of food in front of her.**

Toddlers with Infantile Anorexia not only have problems with recognizing hunger but also a tendency to stop eating when they have eaten only a few bites and the edge of their hunger is taken off. By offering only small amounts of food, the parent stays involved with the toddler without being intrusive, and the toddler is encouraged to eat until full rather than being expected to eat until the jar or the plate is empty.

3. **The parents are encouraged to keep the toddler in the high chair until "mommy's or daddy's tummy is full."** *Children with Infantile Anorexia do not learn to eat until they are full until they learn to sit at the table long enough to eat until fullness.*

Parents cannot and should not make a child eat what they consider the right amount of food because the child has to learn to recognize his internal signals of fullness. However, parents can and should make the child sit at the table until everyone has finished eating. Most toddlers with Infantile Anorexia do not like to sit in the high chair and often protest when they are placed in the chair or try to climb out of it as soon as they can. When they get a little older and are placed on a regular chair, they get off the chair after a few minutes and start running around the room. Older children who have learned some table manners ask to be excused from sitting at the table because they are "bored with eating" and have more interesting things to do.

Toddlers who struggle when being put in the high chair can be given a toy to play with for a few minutes before the meal, but the toy should be removed when the food is put on the tray. Young toddlers under 18 months should be strapped in the high chair, but if they still try to climb out, they should be told in a firm voice that "you need to stay in the chair." If that is not enough, they should be given a time-out by the parent either turning away for 30 seconds or turning the high chair around so that the toddler faces away from the parent. Most toddlers older than 18 months and preschool children who do not stay seated understand when they misbehave and can be given the special time-out described on page 46. Older preschool and school-age children can be taught to stay seated at the table by positive reinforcement and if necessary by using the time-out as well. The children earn a sticker for remaining seated and will get a small reward in the form of a toy when they have earned 10 stickers. When they earn 50 stickers, they will be given a big reward, like going to the zoo or to an amusement park, or having a friend for a sleepover. By this time, the children have gotten used to sitting at the table and have accepted that this is expected from them.

4. Meals should last no longer than 20 to 30 minutes.

Most toddlers can eat adequate amounts of food in about 20 minutes. However, some toddlers with Infantile Anorexia are slow eaters and may need 30 minutes to eat until fullness. The parents should try to adjust their own eating to the pace of the child's eating. However, there is no need to go beyond 30 minutes of mealtime, as sometimes happens when parents hope that their child may take one more bite if they wait a little longer. Children learn to increase their pace of eating if they are hungry enough. However, if the meals take too long, the child will not be hungry for the next meal. Young children do not have any concept of time; consequently, the parents should time their own eating to last 20 to 30 minutes. Children with Infantile Anorexia want to get out of the chair as soon as they have had a few bites of food. However, once they have learned to accept that they have to sit at the table until everybody's "tummy is full" they tend to start eating again and learn to eat until full. It is also important to talk about "the tummy being full" versus "being done," because talking about being full directs the attention of the child to the feeling in his stomach, whereas a child can "be done" for all kinds of reasons, including not liking the food or having something more interesting to do.

5. The parents should not praise or criticize the toddler for how much or how little the toddler is eating.

For the toddler to learn to eat in accord with hunger and fullness, his eating should not be a performance to please or to frustrate his parents. However, to keep the toddler focused and interested in eating, the parents are to encourage self-feeding by offering a second spoon and finger food, and praise the toddler for self-feeding such as by saying, "You used your spoon! Good job!"

6. During feeding, there should not be any toys or television to distract the child.

When children are distracted, they do not pay attention to their inner signals of hunger or fullness. Children who enjoy food tend to overeat, and children who have a low hunger drive forget to eat when they are mesmerized by what they see on television. Parents often resort to distractions when the children are young because infants become so distracted that they do not notice when the parents slip food into their mouth. Consequently, the parents rely on distractions as a way to feed their children. They need to understand that this will interfere with the child's internal regulation, and they need to be helped to give up trying to distract the child.

7. Food is not to be used as a reward or as an expression of the parents' affection.

As Leann Birch (1999) has demonstrated in her research, preschool children can be trained to develop strong likes for sweet desserts, if they have to eat the healthy food first before they are given the dessert, whereas if the dessert food is offered along with the healthy food, the children do not care for the dessert food any more than for the regular meal. Our society has developed some customs that seem to train children to consider sweets, such as candy, cookies, cake, and ice cream, not as food but as treats and as symbols of love and affection by their parents or friends. They develop strong preferences for these foods not only because of the sweet taste but also because of the added sweetness of their symbolic meaning. The associations between these sweet foods and affection are very powerful, and when children get older and long for affection, these foods become the replacement for the love and affection they are missing. A young teenager with Bulimia Nervosa explained her binging on ice cream in the following way: "When I was young, all the affection I got from my parents was associated with special food. My father would take me to the ice-cream parlor for a special treat; my mother would reward me with special foods if I had done well in school. However, now my parents have hardly any time for me anymore, but the food is always there."

8. There should not be any throwing of food or feeding utensils, and older toddlers should be discouraged from playing with the food instead of eating it.

When infants get around 9 months of age, they begin to work on understanding what happens when objects or people disappear out of their sight. Infants experience distress when their primary caretakers disappear, and this is often the age of intense stranger anxiety. We help infants to learn that people or objects do not disappear forever when they cannot be seen by playing peek-a-boo and hide-and-seek. This is also the age when infants like to drop food from the tray of their high chair and look where it went. This behavior needs to be differentiated from an infant or toddler throwing food or feeding utensils because he does not want to eat. As described earlier, infants and toddlers with Infantile Anorexia do not seem to experience much hunger and get easily bored when sitting in the high chair. They play with the food and feeding utensils instead of eating, and when frustrated they throw everything that is in front of them. Consequently, it is helpful to engage the infant in the feeding process by offering a second spoon and encouraging early self-feeding. It is also important to give the toddler just a little bit of food at the time to keep the feeding experience interesting. However, if in spite of these accommodations, the toddler misbehaves and throws food and feeding utensils, he should be given time-out, as described on page 46.

9. Older toddlers and preschool and school-age children should be refocused when they engage in distracting conversations during mealtimes.

Older toddlers and preschool and school-age children with Infantile Anorexia often enjoy talking during mealtime and forget to eat. This can be a real challenge for the parents because if they remain unresponsive to the child's bids for attention, some of these children create their own distractions. The mother of one 3-year-old had been told not to engage in such stimulating conversations with her daughter during mealtime and so sat very quietly with her daughter during the meal; when she gave her daughter a banana to eat, the daughter took the banana and turned it into her friend. While she marched the banana in front of her, she said, "Mammi is not talking to me today, so I will be talking to you, because you are now my friend." A 7-year-old very bright and talkative girl with Infantile Anorexia, when asked why she would not eat when her parents took her out to restaurants with friends of the family, explained to the therapist that "my mouth just feels like talking." Parents need to walk a fine line between being engaged with the child and not being too stimulating, and at times they need to help the child refocus on eating by saying something like "We need to eat now and let's talk later." Most of these children crave parental attention, and setting up a special time of 15 to 30 minutes at some point of the day, when one or the other parent has a "playtime or talking time" with the child, often helps the child to separate mealtimes from playtimes and talking times.

The Time-Out Procedure

In order for the parents to deal successfully with the toddler's behaviors and to set appropriate limits, they are encouraged to use a time-out procedure. This will help the toddler to calm himself when he is upset because he cannot have his way. Self-calming is often very difficult for these toddlers, but at the same time, it is critical for them to learn because of their emotional intensity. Toddlers with Infantile Anorexia tend to be very strong willed and become severely distressed if they cannot have their way. They become very dependent on their parents to help them feel better because they do not know how to calm themselves. Many mothers are so anxious about their toddler's poor eating that they do anything to help their child, and consequently, they often give in to the child and end up being controlled by the child; as one mother put it so pointedly, "I need help. I have a 2-year-old executive in my house."

The time-out procedure was developed to help parents regain control, set appropriate limits, and help their child deal with frustration, learn self-calming, and develop inner controls. Children feel more confident and independent once they have learned to calm themselves. After having gone over the feeding guidelines, the therapist needs to explain the time-out procedure in detail. Without appropriate limit setting, these toddlers do not learn to regulate their eating according to hunger and fullness because their emotions get in the way. It is very important that both parents participate in this treatment session, because children with Infantile Anorexia are exceptionally perceptive and quickly recognize if one parent is not on board.

The time-out procedure has several key elements that need to be explained:

*The parents are to give **only one** warning.* Parents have different thresholds before reacting to their child when she misbehaves. Some parents go through three warnings, and some may go up to five warnings until their patience is exhausted and they become angry and frustrated that the child has not been listening to them. Children learn from observation of their parents' facial expression and tone of voice whether the parent is on the last warning or has a few more rounds to go before acting. Because parents tend to have a consistent pattern of warnings, whether it involves two or three or five, children do not comply until the parent has reached her or his usual last warning. By this time, the parent feels upset and angry because the child has pushed the parent to the point of frustration. The child has effectively trained the parent to go through these cycles of warnings each time there is a conflict. This pattern is very destructive to the parent–child relationship. Consequently, the parents should be encouraged to train themselves to give *one* firm warning and then act by putting the child in time-out.

The child should be put in time-out out in a safe place, where the child is alone and does not see the parents (e.g., the crib, the playpen, a gated room, or, for preschool and older children, the bedroom). Most children with Infantile Anorexia are very willful and become intensely distressed when they are put in time-out the first time. They will not stay in the corner or in an open area, and they will battle with the parents because they want to come out. For toddlers, the crib or playpen works well because the child is safe, and the primary purpose of the time-out is for the child to learn self-calming and self-control. Parents often express concern that the child will have bad associations when taking the time-out in these places, and they fear that it may affect the child's sleep. This time-out procedure is not punitive, and a child knows the difference when he is put in the crib for self-calming or to be punished. Preschool and older children can take the time-out in their room, as long as they are safe. If they do not stay in the room, the lock of their room should be reversed, so that that the door can be locked from outside. The child can be given the choice of the door being unlocked if he stays in the room. Most children quickly opt to stay in the room when they realize that they will be locked in otherwise. The children run in and out of the room and do not settle when the door is unlocked. If the parents have to hold the door closed to keep the child inside the room a struggle ensues and the child will not calm himself. When the child learns that the door will be locked, he will stop trying to get out. Some parents report that once the children have learned to calm themselves in their room, they take a time-out on their own and go to their room to calm themselves when they feel that they are losing control.

The time-out begins only after the child has calmed herself. Initially, when children are taken to their crib or room for time-out, they tend to be very distressed and cry loudly in hopes that the parents will come and rescue them. The first time, the child's distress can last anywhere from 10 minutes to 30 minutes, and some children can carry on for hours before they settle. Once the parents have put the child in time-out, it is very important that they do not break down and take her out before she has calmed. Otherwise, the child will have learned that if she cries loudly enough, the parents will come to her rescue, and the next time she will cry even louder. However, once the child is quiet for a couple of minutes, the parents are to go in and tell the child, "I know it was very hard, but you calmed yourself, and I am very proud that you can calm yourself."

They should continue by saying, "Now, I want you to stay calm and think about what you did wrong. I am setting the timer, and when the alarm goes off, I will come and take you back." Only when the child is calm can she think about what she did wrong. The parent sets the timer for a few minutes for the time-out to begin and leaves the child. Some children still feel angry for being put in time-out and start crying again. In that case, the parent has to go back and stop the timer, and tell the child that the timer will not start until the child has calmed again. When the child is calm again, the parent goes back and says, "I am glad that you calmed yourself, and I am setting the timer again." When the timer goes off, the parent returns, praises her for staying calm, and takes her out of time-out and back to the "scene of the crime."

The child is taken back to correct her behavior. It is very important that the child has to return and correct the behavior, otherwise she has not learned anything from the time-out. Many toddlers with Infantile Anorexia get their first time-out for getting up from the high chair, and they need to return to the high chair and sit until "Mommy's and Daddy's tummies are full." The parents are encouraged to eat for a few more minutes, and the toddler may eat some, but may also just sit there and watch her parents eat. This is all right because the purpose of the time-out was to teach the toddler to sit in the high chair until her parents tell her that she can get up.

However, there are some very strong-willed children who come back and repeat the same unacceptable behavior that got them into time-out before. The parents need to take these children back and repeat the time-out until the child complies with what she was to do. Most children get the idea and correct their behavior after the first time-out. However, there are some children who go through repeated time-outs until they realize that they are not going to win this battle. Once the parents have started the time-out, they need to follow through until the child complies. The child cannot win this battle. Otherwise, the child will continue to control the parents.

The first time-out can be very difficult for the child and the parents, and it may take a few hours until the child learns to calm down and gain self-control. Because the first time-out can be very time consuming and stressful for the parents, it is important that the parents plan it for a weekend day, when both parents can be at home, have nothing on their schedule, and can do it together. It is also important that they explain to the child the different steps of the time-out procedure before the first implementation, so the child knows what to expect.

The handouts that follow show the feeding guidelines and the time-out procedural steps. With these, parents can follow the therapist step-by-step in learning how to work with their child, and they can take the handouts home to refresh their memory. However, the guidelines should not be given to the parents without explanations. The parents need to understand the rationale behind the different instructions, and the therapist needs to individualize the guidelines to adjust to the special needs of the child and his parents.

FEEDING GUIDELINES

Irene Chatoor, MD

FOR TEACHING YOUR CHILD HOW TO REGULATE EATING ACCORDING TO HUNGER AND FULLNESS

- To help your child feel hungry, feed your child at regular times and space meals and snacks 3–4 hours apart.

  – Do not allow your child to have any snacks, juice, or milk between scheduled meal and snack times. If your child gets thirsty, offer only water.

- Serve small portions and allow your child to ask for second, third, and fourth helpings. This will help your child be engaged in the eating process and prevent your child from being bored or overwhelmed by large amounts of food.

  – Most important, it will help your child to learn to eat until full.

- Teach your child to sit at the table until "Mommy's and Daddy's tummies are full."

  – Children do not learn to eat until they are full until they learn to sit at the table long enough to eat until fullness.

- Do not offer more than three different foods at any one meal and remain seated at the table with your child.

- Meals should last no longer than 20 to 30 minutes, even if your child has eaten very little or nothing. Your child will learn to make up for the minimal food intake at the next meal.

- Praise your child for self-feeding skills, but keep a neutral attitude about your child's food intake.

Continued

– Do not praise or criticize your child for how much or how little she eats.

– Your child's eating is not a performance, but should be regulated internally by your child's physiological needs.

• Do not allow any distractions (e.g., toys, books, television) during meals or snacks.

– When distracted, children do not pay attention to their inner signals of hunger and fullness.

• Do not use food as a present, as a reward, for comfort, or as an expression of your affection.

– Do not place emphasis on sweets and candy; ask your child whether he wants to eat the dessert or the other foods first.

• Discourage your child from playing with the food or talking too much instead of eating during mealtime. Have a special playtime or talking time outside of mealtime.

• If your child gets up from the chair, throws food or feeding utensils, or misbehaves in other ways, give her ONE warning. If she does not stop the behavior, give her a time-out.

TIME-OUT OUTLINE

Irene Chatoor, MD

TO HELP YOUNG CHILDREN TO ACCEPT LIMITS, TO CALM THEMSELVES AND GAIN SELF-CONTROL

- When your child misbehaves, give him only *one* warning!

- If your child does not listen, put him in time-out in his crib, playpen, a gated-off room, or his bedroom, where the child is safe, alone, and not able to see you.

- If your child cries, wait until he has calmed. Do not interact with your child while he is crying or talking to you. The time-out begins only after your child has calmed himself.

- After he has calmed himself, go in and tell your child that you understand that it was very difficult for him to calm himself, that you are proud of him for calming himself, and that you want him to stay calm and think about what he did wrong.

- Then set the alarm of your time-out clock (about 1 minute for each year of your child's life) and tell your child to stay calm, that you will be back when the alarm goes off.

- After the alarm has gone off, praise your child again for staying calm and take him back to the "scene of the crime."

- Ask your child to correct his behavior (e.g., "Show Mommy how you sit nicely in your chair while we are eating").

- If your child is still angry and misbehaves again, repeat the time-out procedure until your child complies.

IMPORTANT

- Do not take your child out of time-out when he is crying.
- Do not stop the time-out procedures until your child complies.
- Pick your battles with your child, but make sure that you win!
- Explain the time-out prodedure to your child when he is calm before you apply it the first time.

These therapeutic steps—addressing the toddler's temperament, helping the parents understand their difficulties in setting limits, and providing them with specific guidelines on how to structure mealtimes in order to facilitate the toddler's internal regulation of eating and how to use the time-out procedure to set limits on the toddler's behaviors that interfere with eating—can be best accomplished in two or three double sessions. Meeting with the parents for 2 hours at a time allows for more intensive discussions and promotes a better therapeutic alliance. Once the parents have received the feeding guidelines, they usually like to have a few weeks to practice with their child and then come back to review the feeding and discuss what seems to help and where they have run into difficulties. Some parents observe major behavioral changes and improved food intake by the toddler within weeks. Other children move more gradually and need months before they show better awareness of their hunger feelings and learn to eat until they are satiated. When the children eat more, they gain weight at a better rate, and then, after a month or two, show a pickup in their linear growth. However, when children with Infantile Anorexia experience more excitement, such as from a birthday party, house guests, or travel, they tend to lose their appetite and may revert to eating very little again. Once the excitement is over, they usually settle and regain their appetite. This is important for the parents to be aware of, so that they do not become panicked, thinking that the child is back to where he or she started before the treatment. In general, the conflict over eating between parents and child can be neutralized by this intervention, and often the parents experience great relief and enjoy their children more fully.

The following case illustrates the development of symptoms, the assessment by our Multidisciplinary Feeding Disorders Team, and the treatment to facilitate internal regulation of eating in a toddler with Infantile Anorexia:

Example: John was a 20-month-old Caucasian male, the first child of highly educated parents, who both had been working in their professions before his birth, but John's mother, Mrs. Hardman, stayed home after John was born. John was referred by his pediatrician for an evaluation by the Multidisciplinary Feeding Disorders Team because of food refusal and poor weight gain. John had never been a good eater, but his appetite had worsened during the last several months since he had learned to walk. He often did not want to go in the high chair or tried to climb out of the high chair after he had eaten a few bites of food. His parents reported that he never asked for food, and it was very difficult to tell when he was hungry. He ate a fairly wide variety of foods, although his food preferences varied from day to day. John's parents offered him food several times throughout the day and let him drink milk from a sippy cup whenever he wanted some, but generally, he would just take a little and then refuse to eat or drink anymore.

John was born full-term, weighing 9 pounds. Feeding was an issue from the beginning. He slept through feedings early on and needed to be awakened to nurse. When John was awake, if somebody would enter the room, he would stop feeding and look around. He rarely cried for food, so he was placed on a schedule and offered the breast at regular intervals. At 6 months of age, cereal was offered and then baby foods, which he accepted well but ate very small amounts. At 8 months, finger foods were introduced, which he seemed to enjoy, but again in small amounts. At 12 months old, he advanced to a wide variety of table foods, which he enjoyed eating. At this age, he started to make his first steps and became increasingly busy, "getting into everything." He started to resist going into the high chair and had to be coaxed by his parents with toys that they placed on the tray of the chair. With further distractions, John would eat a few bites, but then become restless and try to climb out of the high chair. Once Mr. and Mrs. Hardman let him out, he would run around the room, and they would follow him with the spoon to get some more food into him. At 14 months of age, he was weaned off the breast. He initially refused to drink milk out of the sippy cup, but after the milk was mixed with water, over time John accepted the milk without difficulty.

His past medical history and his physical examination were unremarkable. His nutritional assessment placed his height at the 5th percentile and his weight below the 5th percentile for his age. His weight for height was below the 5th percentile, which was calculated at 80% of ideal body weight. However, his head circumference was at the 20th percentile. In reviewing his growth chart, it was apparent that there was slight deceleration in weight gain starting between 3 and 6 months, with further deceleration from the 25th percentile to between the 5th and 10th percentile between 6 and 12 months, and further deceleration to below the 5th percentile starting at 12 months of age. His linear growth fell to the 25th percentile between 8 and 12 months of age and decelerated further to the 5th percentile starting at 12 months of age. There was an obvious lag of a few months between the deceleration of height compared to the deceleration of his weight.

The analysis of a 3-day food record that Mrs. Hardman had filled out revealed that on average, John was eating 60% of the daily recommended allowance for a child of his age, but that 50% of his calories were coming from milk enriched with calories, vitamins, zinc, and iron, which the pediatrician had recommended a few months ago when John's food refusal and poor growth became more and more entrenched.

The oral motor assessment found that John's oral motor skills appeared age-appropriate and were not a limitation to his feeding. A developmental assessment found that John's cognitive and general motor skills were in the high average range.

The observation of John and his mother during feeding and play from behind a one-way mirror, a part of the psychiatric assessment, revealed that John was resistant to going into the high chair but settled when his mother lured him with a toy. He took a few bites of the food in front of him but started to look around the room, pointing to a wall hanging with trains, noticed the clock on the wall, and stopped eating. When his mother tried to feed him some yogurt with the spoon, he batted the spoon away and tried to get up from the high chair. His mother tried to draw his attention to another toy she had kept in reserve, and he settled back in the high chair temporarily. However, the novelty wore off quickly. John refused to eat any more food and pushed the plate with the food in front of him off the tray onto the floor. His mother looked defeated, took him out of the high chair and allowed him to run around the room. She approached him a few times with some finger food, but John was too busy exploring the room to pay any attention to his mother's food.

In contrast to the feeding, during play, John and his mother were engaged in give-and-take interactions and seemed to enjoy each other.

The interview of the parents revealed that Mrs. Hardman had been a poor eater as a child, that she had been small and thin all through childhood, and that she grew up to be the smallest of her family. She only gained some more weight and started to fill in during and after her pregnancy with John. She admitted that she often forgot to eat when she got very busy and that she could not eat when stressed. Her family often compared her to her grandmother, who, she was told, had been seen in all of the pediatric hospitals of the major European cities by the time she was 8 years old, because she had been so thin and fragile. The father professed that he had a good appetite and reported that he had always been tall and athletic. However, one of his sisters was a picky eater as a child and developed Anorexia Nervosa as a young adult. Both parents were worried that John would grow up to be a thin little boy, and the mother confessed that sometimes, if John had eaten hardly anything during the day, she could not sleep and would worry that he would die.

The parents had waited to have children because of their careers, and then they had difficulty conceiving for several years. They both had good relations with their own parents who lived in other cities, several hours away, and visited only occasionally. However, the parents had a good social network in the area.

After the evaluation, the team consisting of a nurse practitioner who served as the coordinator of the team, a gastroenterologist, a nutritionist, an occupational therapist, and the psychiatrist met with the parents and presented their findings. The gastroenterologist explained that John was physically healthy, and the occupational therapist described that he had good oral motor functioning, including a rotary chew (moving the food from the front of his mouth to the side and chewing it), and that there were no limitations to his eating from an oral motor point of view. The nutritionist described John's deceleration of growth, which became most marked after 12 months of age, and pointed out that his head growth had continued to progress at a normal rate. She explained that John's nutritional intake was lower than expected for a child of his age, but that with the help of the enriched formula, he was getting all the essential micronutrients. Finally, the psychiatrist described John as a bright little boy who seemed too busy exploring the world to pay attention to his inner signals of hunger, and consequently, he did not want to be interrupted in his play activities and be confined to the high chair. She explained to the parents that the therapeutic challenge was to help John to become aware of his hunger signals and learn to sit in the high chair until his tummy was full. The consensus of the team was that John was not in any nutritional danger, and that the psychiatrist would take over the intervention.

The parents were invited back to meet with the psychiatrist for 2 hours, without John, to go over the feeding guidelines and the time-out procedure. The psychiatrist helped Mr. and Mrs. Hardman to develop a daily schedule of meals that were spaced 3–4 hours apart to allow John to feel hungry. Mr. Hardman had been coming home late and was eating after the mother had tried to feed John, but he committed to make an effort to be home by 6:30 p.m. in order to have a "family dinner." Mrs. Hardman struggled with giving up the distractions she had used to get John to eat and was anxious when asked to deny John food in between the scheduled meals and the afternoon snack. The father seemed more comfortable with setting limits for John, and the couple decided to begin implementing the feeding guidelines and time-out procedure on the weekend, when both parents were at home and could support each other. The major issue was to get John into the high chair and to keep him there "until Mommy's and Daddy's tummies were full." It was decided that this was a likely issue that would come up, and that John would get his first time-out to teach him that he had to sit in the high chair. The father accepted the role of implementing the first time-out and taking John to his crib in the bedroom. Mr. and Mrs. Hardman wanted to come back without John in 3 weeks to discuss how far they had gotten in implementing the changes they had agreed upon.

John's parents reported back that John had been very distressed when given his first time-out and that it had taken him more than half an hour to calm himself, but that once he calmed and later returned to the high chair, he sat quietly without any further effort to get out and even took a few bites of the food in front of him. They were surprised that after that dramatic first time-out, he willingly went into the high chair and did not challenge them anymore by trying to get out. John seemed to feel hungry some of the meals, but usually had a good meal followed by eating not much during the next meal. Overall, his food intake had improved, and he was calmer during the meals. The parents found giving him just a small portion of food at a time very helpful because he seemed to stay interested in the food. Mr. Hardman admitted that he actually had started to look forward to coming home in the evening and having a family meal.

A month later, John and his parents returned for a family meal in the office, and the psychiatrist observed them from behind a one-way mirror. John went willingly into the high chair and seemed hungry initially, but after about 5 minutes, he stopped eating, looked at the pictures on the wall, tried to draw his parents' attention to the microphone on the ceiling, and seemed to forget to eat. The parents responded to his curiosity and soon were engaged in a conversation about the things that John had observed and talked about. In the meantime, John had lost interest in his food, and mealtime was over. In the discussion with John's parents, the psychiatrist pointed out how tempting it was to be seduced by John's curiosity, and they were encouraged to refocus him on eating and set up a playtime and talking time after dinner, so that they could tell him, "Let's eat now, and later we will talk." The psychiatrist also made them aware that they could expect that John would respond to more exciting events in their lives, such as house guests, birthday parties, or travel, by "losing his appetite," and that after these events, he most likely would eat better again. Overall, the parents were encouraged by the progress they had made in helping John respond to his inner signals of hunger and fullness.

During the last follow-up, when John was 2½ years old, he was eating better during most of the meals, he was off the enriched formula, getting most of his calories from table food, and he was drinking regular milk at mealtimes. He had gained weight and grown a few inches, which placed him on the 5th percentile for weight and the 10th percentile for height. Mr. and Mrs. Hardman reported that they had very enjoyable dinners together with John, and that they were thinking of having another baby.

Use of Dietary Supplements and Medication in Treatment

Some infants and toddlers with Infantile Anorexia eat very little but continue to nurse or drink from the bottle, which is often their primary source of nutritional intake. Most of the toddlers with Infantile Anorexia appear to use these feedings more for comfort than to fill their little stomachs, and consequently, they usually drink only small amounts of milk at a time. Although in the second year of life, toddlers are usually transitioned to regular cow's milk, pediatricians like to optimize the nutritional intake of children with Infantile Anorexia by recommending formulas that are enriched with calories, vitamins, and minerals. These formulas are helpful in supporting the children's nutrition until they learn to eat more food that provides them with the necessary nutrients. They serve as a safety net and relieve some of the parents' anxiety so that they can work with the therapist on helping their toddler learn to eat more table food. However, the drinking of formula needs to be incorporated into the meal schedule; otherwise, the toddler will not be hungry at mealtime. Once the child is eating better, she can be gradually weaned from the supplemental formula.

There are some children whose behavior around mealtime improves, who learn to sit at the table until their parents have finished eating, but who continue to eat very little and grow poorly. For these children, medication may be helpful to stimulate their appetite. Cyproheptadine is a medication used for treating allergy symptoms that was found to also have an appetite-stimulating effect. Its action is through blocking histamine and serotonin.

Early studies by Halmi, Eckert, LaDu, and Cohen (1986) with adolescents and young adults with Anorexia Nervosa demonstrated that cyproheptadine resulted in a greater increase of weight and greater decrease in depression when compared with placebo. No studies using cyproheptadine with young children have been published. However, cyproheptadine is often prescribed by pediatricians and gastroenterologists to increase toddlers' appetite. In most children, cyproheptadine results in an immediate increase in appetite, and this effect may last for 2 or 3 weeks, when the child's appetite decreases again, although the appetite may not be as poor as it was before the introduction of the medication. When the medication is stopped for a week or two and reintroduced, the child's appetite may pick up again, and this may last for another 2 to 3 weeks. Consequently, some physicians use cyproheptadine in cycles of 2 weeks on and 1 or 2 weeks off, or 4 days on and 3 days off, to help the child get into a better eating pattern. The medication is generally well tolerated, and the parents experience great relief when they see their child eating. However, this medication does not cure the problem; some children respond only initially, and the medication should not be a substitute for using the feeding guidelines to facilitate internal regulation of eating.

Differential Diagnosis and Comorbidities

Infantile Anorexia is frequently associated with Sensory Food Aversions, which are described in chapter 5. Both feeding disorders are characterized by food refusal. However, whereas children with Infantile Anorexia have a poor appetite and may refuse a food one day and eat it the next day, children with Sensory Food Aversions consistently refuse certain foods because of their taste, texture, or smell. Children who have Sensory Food Aversions have a good appetite, will readily eat foods with which they are comfortable, and usually have a normal weight. However, if children have a combination of both feeding disorders, they have a poor appetite, they may eat some foods one day and refuse to eat them the next day, and they also consistently refuse certain foods and get very upset if their parents urge them to eat these foods. They may get so upset that they refuse to eat anything. Consequently, these children have very serious eating and growth problems. It is very important to diagnose and treat each feeding disorder that is described in the chapter on complex feeding disorders.

Infantile Anorexia is also frequently associated with sleep disorders. Toddlers with Infantile Anorexia had more irregular feeding and sleep patterns than did healthy eaters, based on ratings by the children's mothers (Chatoor, Hirsch, et al., 1998). In the study by Monaghan and colleagues (2007), almost half of the children with Infantile Anorexia had problems going to sleep or were waking up in the night, not being able to go back to sleep on their own and moving into their parents' bed, or cosleeping with their parents altogether because it was too difficult for the parents to help their children to regulate sleep on their own.

As we learned from our study (Chatoor, Ganiban, et al., 2004), children with Infantile Anorexia tend to have a higher level of physiological arousal and have more difficulty down-regulating their arousal than healthy eaters. This arousal pattern seems to serve them well when they are active and eager to learn, but during mealtime and bedtime when children need to relax and down-regulate their arousal, these children are too "wired" to settle. They become clingy and dependent on their parents to help them calm down. Although some parents establish bedtime routines and set limits to the child's clinging early on, other parents become captives of the child's clinging behavior. These parents need help facilitating the child's self-regulation of sleep, similar to helping their child to develop internal regulation of eating.

As described earlier in this chapter in the Temperament section, children with Infantile Anorexia demonstrate more separation anxiety and may show school phobia when they get older. They are often very intense children who find it difficult to calm themselves when they are upset and who cling to their parents to help them feel better. The clinging behaviors of these children can become very coercive, and some parents find themselves controlled by their child. For these children, the time-out procedure is key to facilitate self-calming and self-reliance.

References

Ammaniti, M., Ambruzzi, A. M., Lucarelli, L., Cimino, S., & D'Olimpio, F. (2004). Malnutrition and dysfunctional mother-child feeding interactions: Clinical assessment and research implications. *Journal of the American College of Nutrition, 23*(3), 259–271.

Ammaniti, M., Cimino, S., Lucarelli, L., Speranza, A. M., & Vismara, L. (2004). Infantile anorexia and the child caregiver relationship: An empirical study on attachment patterns. *Funzione Gamma Journal, 14*, 1–19.

Birch, L. L. (1999). Development of food preferences. *Annual Review of Nutrition, 19*, 41–62.

Chatoor, I. (1989). Infantile anorexia nervosa: A developmental disorder of separation and individuation. *Journal of the American Academy of Psychoanalysis, 17*, 43–64.

Chatoor, I., & Ammaniti, M. (2007). A classification of feeding disorders of infancy and early childhood. In W. E. Narrow, M. B. First, P. Sirovatka, & D. A. Regier (Eds.), *Age and gender considerations in psychiatric diagnosis: A research agenda for DSM-V* (pp. 227–242). Arlington, VA: American Psychiatric Press.

Chatoor, I., & Egan, J. (1983). Nonorganic failure to thrive and dwarfism due to food refusal: A separation disorder. *Journal of the American Academy of Child and Adolescent Psychiatry, 27*, 294–301.

Chatoor, I., Egan, J., Getson, P., Menvielle, E., & O'Donnell, R. (1988). Mother-infant interactions in infantile anorexia nervosa. *Journal of the American Academy of Child and Adolescent Psychiatry, 27*, 535–540.

Chatoor, I., Ganiban, J., Colin, V., Plummer, N., & Harmon, R. (1998). Attachment and feeding problems: A reexamination of non-organic failure to thrive and attachment insecurity. *Journal of the American Academy of Child and Adolescent Psychiatry, 37*, 1217–1224.

Chatoor, I., Ganiban, J., Harrison, J., & Hirsch, R. (2001). Observation of feeding in the diagnosis of posttraumatic feeding disorder of infancy. *Journal of the American Academy of Child and Adolescent Psychiatry, 40*, 595–602.

Chatoor, I., Ganiban, J., Hirsch, R., Borman-Spurrell, E., & Mrazek, D. (2000). Maternal characteristics and toddler temperament in infantile anorexia. *Journal of the American Academy of Child and Adolescent Psychiatry, 39*, 743–751.

Chatoor, I., Ganiban, J., Surles, J., & Doussard-Roosevelt, J. (2004). Physiological regulation in infantile anorexia: A pilot study. *Journal of the American Academy of Child and Adolescent Psychiatry, 43*, 1019–1025.

Chatoor, I., Getson, P., Menvielle, E., O'Donnell, R., Rivera, Y., Brasseaux, C., et al. (1997). A feeding scale for research and clinical practice to assess mother-infant interactions in the first three years of life. *Infant Mental Health Journal, 18*, 76–91.

Chatoor, I., Hirsch R., Ganiban, J., Persinger, M., & Hamburger, E. (1998). Diagnosing infantile anorexia: The observation of mother infant interactions. *Journal of the American Academy of Child and Adolescent Psychiatry, 37*, 959–967.

Chatoor, I., Hirsch, R., & Persinger, M. (1997). Facilitating internal regulation of eating: A treatment model for infantile anorexia. *Infants and Young Children, 9*, 12–22.

Chatoor, I., Kerzner, B., Zorc, L., Persinger, M., Simenson, R., & Mrazek, D. (1992). Two year old twins refuse to eat: A multidisciplinary approach to diagnosis and treatment. *Infant Mental Health Journal, 13*, 252–268.

Chatoor, I., Surles, J., Ganiban, J., Beker, L., McWade Paez, L., & Kerzner, B. (2004). Failure to thrive and cognitive development in toddlers with infantile anorexia. *Pediatrics, 113*, e440–e447.

Dahl, M. (1987). Early feeding problems in an affluent society: III. Follow-up at two years: Natural course, health, behaviour and development. *Acta Paediatrica Scandinavica, 76*, 872–880.

Dahl, M., Rydell, A. M., & Sundelin, C. (1994). Children with early refusal to eat: Follow-up during primary school. *Acta Paediatrica Scandinavica, 83*, 54–58.

Halmi, K. A., Eckert, E., LaDu, T. J., & Cohen, J. (1986). Anorexia nervosa. Treatment efficacy of cyproheptadine and amitriptyline. *Archives of General Psychiatry, 43*, 177–181.

Kotler, L. A., Cohen, P., Davies, M., Pine, D. S., & Walsh, B. T. (2001). Longitudinal relationships between childhood, adolescent, and adult eating disorders. *Journal of the American Academy of Child and Adolescent Psychiatry, 40*, 1434–1440.

Lucarelli, L., Ambruzzi, A. M., Cimino, S., D'Olimpio, F., & Finistrella, V. (2003). Feeding disorders in infancy: An empirical study on mother-infant interactions. *Minerva Pediatrica, 55*, 243–259.

Lucarelli, L., Cimino, S., Petrocchi, M., & Ammaniti, M. (2007, October). *Infantile anorexia: A longitudinal study on maternal and child psychopathology.* Abstract presented at Eating Disorders Research Society, Pittsburgh, PA.

Marchi, M., & Cohen, P. (1990). Early childhood eating behaviors and adolescent eating disorders. *Journal of the American Academy of Child and Adolescent Psychiatry, 29*, 112–117.

Monaghan, M., Lewin, D., Hahn, A., Ganiban, J., Morar, V., Brinkmeier, L., & Chatoor, I. (2007). Sleep characteristics of toddlers with infantile anorexia. *Sleep, 30*, A97.

Narrow, W. E., First, M. B., Sirovatka, P., & Regier, D. A. (Eds.). (2007). *Age and gender considerations in psychiatric diagnosis: A research agenda for DSM-V.* Arlington, VA: American Psychiatric Press.

Scheeringa, M., Anders, T., Boris, N., Carter, A., Chatoor, I., Egger, H., et al. (2003). Research diagnostic criteria for infants and preschool children: The process and empirical support. *Journal of the American Academy of Child and Adolescent Psychiatry, 42*, 1504–1512.

Waterlow, J. C., Buzina, R., Keller, W., Lan, J. M., Nichaman, M. Z., & Tanner, J. M. (1977). The presentation and use of height and weight data for comparing the nutritional status of groups of children under the age of 10 years. *Bulletin of the World Health Organization, 55*, 489–498.

ZERO TO THREE. (2005). *Diagnostic classification of mental health and developmental disorders of infancy and early childhood: Revised edition. (DC:0–3R).* Washington, DC: Author.

5

SENSORY FOOD AVERSIONS

Nosology

DIFFERENT ASPECTS of Sensory Food Aversions have been described by various names. Most commonly, children with Sensory Food Aversions are considered "picky eaters," "selective eaters," or "choosy eaters." Some authors refer to the refusal to eat certain foods as "food aversion" and to the fear of trying new foods as "food neophobia." I chose to describe this feeding disorder as Sensory Food Aversions because the children experience specific foods as strongly aversive in taste, texture, temperature, or smell, and they frequently have other sensory difficulties as well. Their aversive reactions can range from grimacing or spitting out the food to gagging and vomiting. After an initial aversive reaction, the children usually refuse to continue eating that particular food and often refuse to try other foods that seem to remind them of foods which triggered aversive reactions. I will review some of the related literature that has addressed symptoms of Sensory Food Aversions.

The term *picky eater* has not been well defined and is used by different authors to mean different things. Marchi and Cohen (1990) defined picky eating by the presence of three of the following child behaviors: does not eat enough, is often or very often choosy about food, usually eats slowly, or is usually not interested in food. The authors found that picky eating in early childhood predicted symptoms of Anorexia Nervosa during adolescence. However, "does not eat enough" and "is not interested in food," according to the classification in this book, are symptoms of Infantile Anorexia, and "is often or very often choosy about food" would be considered a symptom of Sensory Food Aversions. As I will discuss later, children can be comorbid for Infantile Anorexia and Sensory Food Aversions.

Accordingly, the children in the study by Marchi and Cohen may have presented with symptoms of Infantile Anorexia or Sensory Food Aversions, or they may have had symptoms of both feeding disorders. This makes it hard to interpret from this study whether Infantile Anorexia, Sensory Food Aversions, or both are posing risk factors for Anorexia Nervosa.

A more recent study by Carruth, Ziegler, Gordon, and Barr (2004) on the prevalence of picky eating among a national random sample of more than 3,000 infants and toddlers used telephone interviews to ask parents whether they considered their child a very picky eater, a somewhat picky eater, or not a picky eater. The meaning of picky eating was not defined by the interviewer. Then the data of the toddlers described by their parents as "very picky eaters" and "somewhat picky eaters" were combined to form one "picky eater" data set. The authors found that the prevalence of picky eaters consistently increased for both sexes between 4 and 24 months, ranging from 17% to 47% for males and 23% to 54% for females. They reported that the age groups of 7 to 8 months and 9 to 11 months had 17 statistically significant differences in energy and nutrient intake associated with picky eater status, whereas intakes for all the other age groupings had only 6 statistically significant differences. However, for all nutrients, mean intakes were well above the recommended dietary allowances or adequate intakes for picky and nonpicky eater groups. These data give some interesting information on the high prevalence of what parents experience as picky eating of their young children, most notably for children between the ages of 4 and 24 months. However, because the authors combined "somewhat picky" and "very picky eaters," the nutritional data are not very helpful because they cover the whole range of picky eaters and do not identify children for whom the picky eating may be associated with serious dietary deficiencies.

A review article by Dovey, Staples, Gibson, and Halford (2007) stated that "picky/fussy" eaters are usually defined as children who consume an inadequate variety of foods through rejection of a substantial amount of foods that are familiar (as well as unfamiliar) to them, whereas food neophobia is generally regarded as the reluctance to eat new foods or the avoidance of new foods. The authors saw food neophobia and picky/fussy eating as related constructs that are theoretically and behaviorally different. They saw neophobia as a part of picky/fussy eating but not accounting for the entire behavioral profile of the picky/fussy eater.

Timimi, Douglas, and Tsiftsopoulou (1997) described case studies of "selective eaters" ranging in age from 4 to 14 years. They defined selective eating as a specific and persistent pattern of behavior consisting of refusal to eat any foods outside of a limited range of preferred foods, and they described accompanying behaviors that include resisting attempts at self-feeding, gagging, spitting out food, mealtime disruptive behaviors, playing with food at mealtimes, excessively slow eating, and difficulties swallowing or chewing food. These authors also observed heightened anxiety, obsessive compulsive symptoms (both food- and non-food-related), and frequent social and school difficulties in these children. Their description of "selective eaters" fit the picture of children with Sensory Food Aversions.

Rydell, Dahl, and Sundelin (1995) described "choosy eaters" as children who show choosiness, manifested in refusal of foods, eating little, and disinterest in food. Similar to Marchi and Cohen (1990), they combined selective eating with eating little and disinterest in food, symptoms of Infantile Anorexia.

This brief review of some of the literature demonstrates how poorly defined picky eating and the other terms are and how difficult it is to compare studies because there are no clear definitions for specific feeding disorders. The diagnostic criteria for Sensory Food Aversions, listed below, first describe the typical behaviors that characterize this feeding disorder, followed by criteria for impairment and exclusionary criteria. The criteria for impairment are either in the nutritional area (specific dietary insufficiencies of micronutrients) or involve delay of oral motor and speech development, or are in the child's social–emotional development, and sometimes there is a combination of all three areas. Because the studies on picky eating report very high prevalence rates, it can be assumed that Sensory Food Aversions are quite common in the general population and occur on a continuum, with some children refusing only a few foods and others refusing whole food groups. Therefore, it is important to identify children who have serious feeding problems and differentiate them, through the use of the criteria of impairment, from those who might be little affected by the few foods they cannot tolerate. The diagnostic criteria listed below were included in *Diagnostic Classification of Mental Health and Developmental Disorders of Infancy and Early Childhood: Revised Edition (DC:0–3R;* ZERO TO THREE, 2005) and were described by Chatoor and Ammaniti (2007) in *Age and Gender Considerations in Psychiatric Diagnosis: A Research Agenda for DSM-V* (Narrow, First, Sirovatka, & Regier 2007).

Diagnostic Criteria

A. This feeding disorder is characterized by the infant's or child's consistent refusal to eat certain foods with specific tastes, textures, temperatures, or smells for at least 1 month.

B. The onset of the food refusal occurs during the introduction of a new or different type of food that is aversive to the child (e.g., the child may drink one type of milk but refuse another milk with a different taste; he may eat pureed food but refuse lumpy baby food or solid food that needs to be chewed; he may eat crunchy types of food but refuse purees).

C. The child's reactions to aversive foods range from grimacing or spitting out the food to gagging and vomiting. After an aversive reaction, the child refuses to continue eating the food and frequently generalizes and refuses other foods with a similar color, appearance, or smell. Consequently, the child may refuse whole food groups.

D. The child is reluctant to try unfamiliar new foods but eats without difficulty when offered preferred foods.

E. Without supplementation, the child demonstrates specific dietary deficiencies (i.e., vitamins, iron, zinc, or protein) but usually does not show any growth deficiency and may even be overweight, and/or

- Displays oral motor and expressive speech delay, and/or

- Starting during the preschool years, the child demonstrates anxiety during mealtime and avoids social situations that involve eating.

F. The food refusal does not follow a traumatic event to the oropharynx.

G. Refusal to eat specific foods is not related to food allergies or any other medical illness.

Clinical Presentation

This feeding disorder can become symptomatic as early as the first few weeks of life. Jacobi, Agras, Bryson, and Hammer (2003) reported from a prospective study on children who by parental report and by laboratory measures were picky eaters who ate less of a variety of foods and often avoided vegetables. The authors found that these children exhibited a different sucking pattern during the first month of life. They had more than 100 fewer sucks per feeding session than nonpicky children, and 17% of the picky eaters refused to suck at all. Some mothers of children who were later diagnosed with Sensory Food Aversions have reported that as babies their children did not want to latch on to the breast and that they had to switch them to bottle feedings. These were usually children who seemed to be very sensitive to the texture of food, gagged, and spit out stage 3 baby foods, which are a combination of pureed food with lumps of other food in it. One explanation for the feeding behavior of these infants may be that the irregularity of the nipple of the breast causes more sensory input for the baby than the smooth nipple of the bottle, which is more easily tolerated. Other mothers of children with Sensory Food Aversions reported that even in the first few weeks or months of life, their children would not accept switching to a new formula, that they would cry and refuse to drink the new formula but readily accept switching back to the old formula.

More often, children with Sensory Food Aversions become symptomatic around 6 to 10 months of age when they are introduced to a variety of baby foods, especially stage 3 food. Infants may react to the new taste or texture of baby food by grimacing, spitting out the food or by gagging and vomiting. If the aversive reaction is mild and the infant only grimaces, she may accept the food again and sometimes tolerate it on repeated exposures. However, some infants become very distressed if the parent offers the aversive food again, especially if the food triggered gagging or vomiting. These infants seem to learn by association, and they will watch the parents very closely to see what type of food the parent brings them. They seem to generalize their fear of one food to other foods that may have the same color or consistency, and they begin to reject whole food groups, such as purees or lumpy baby foods or green vegetables. The harder the parents try to get these infants to eat, the more fearful the infants seem to get and the more foods they begin to reject.

Most children begin to show strong reactions to certain foods during the toddler years when they are introduced to a variety of table foods. During this intense developmental period, toddlers struggle with issues of autonomy and dependency, and during each meal, parent and toddler have to negotiate who is going to put the spoon into the toddler's mouth. Once toddlers learn that the parents are very keen to get them to eat, they take control and refuse the food that the parents offer. Often their acceptance or rejection of food depends on their mood and their need to please or their wish to control the parents. Consequently, many toddlers become picky about which food they want to eat and which food they decide to reject. Their choice of foods often changes from meal to meal or from day to day, whereas toddlers with Sensory Food Aversions are more consistent in their food choices, although they are not beyond trying to control their parents by asking for certain foods and then rejecting them. Parents of toddlers with Sensory Food Aversions often do not take it seriously when the toddler initially spits out certain foods or gags on them, and they offer the food again because they believe that the toddler will get used to it. The parents may have heard about the need for repeated exposures to a food until the young child gets used to it, and they keep trying to get their toddler to accept their healthy foods. But then they are faced with a toddler who cries or becomes increasingly stubborn, and they realize that the child will not accept these foods, no matter how hard they coax, beg, or threaten the child. The parents are often told by other family members that they are not strict enough, and they are given advice to offer the child only food that the rest of the family eats, so that when their child is hungry enough, he or she will eat. The parents then find that their child goes for days without eating, and they realize that they have to stop this intervention. As the tension builds during mealtime, the child becomes more anxious and increasingly reluctant to try new foods.

These children may refuse to eat whole food categories, most commonly vegetables, fruits, and meats. In extreme cases they even refuse to eat a preferred food if it touched another food on the plate, if it does not have the right temperature, or if it is not prepared by a specific restaurant or company. The diet of children who refuse to eat vegetables and fruits is often deficient in vitamins, and children who refuse to drink milk or eat meats may not get adequate amounts of protein, zinc, and iron. Many children with Sensory Food Aversions prefer a diet of sugary foods or salty crackers, and some of them become overweight and may develop problems with high cholesterol. In addition, children who refuse to eat foods that require more chewing, such as meats, hard vegetables or fruits, experience delay in oral motor development, which may be associated with articulation difficulties.

The following case illustrates the development of symptoms of Sensory Food Aversions from infancy into the toddler years:

Example: Robert was 19 months old when he was referred for an evaluation by the Multidisciplinary Feeding Disorders Team because of his limited diet and his refusal to try new foods. Some foods, such as eggs and peas, had evoked severe gagging episodes when they touched his tongue, and there had been some isolated episodes of vomiting with foods he did not like, after which he refused to eat many foods. Foods that he would eat included yogurt, American cheese, rice cereal, crackers, cookies, waffles, pancakes, pastas, bananas, and sliced pears. Foods that he refused to eat included meats, poultry, eggs, vegetables, most fruits, and pizza. He also drank a mixture of enriched toddler formula three times a day. His appetite was best in the morning, and he ate least in the evening at family dinner.

Robert's birth history was unremarkable. He was born full-term and weighed 8 pounds and 2 ounces at birth. However, he did not nurse well. He had difficulty latching on and had a nonnutritive suck. Some of these difficulties improved with the help of a lactation consultant, but Mrs. Camp, his mother, had to supplement breast-feeding with formula from the bottle about once or twice a day. At 6 months old, when Robert was introduced to cereal, he did a lot of grimacing, but when his mother mixed the cereal with baby food, he gradually accepted it. He accepted the different tastes of baby food without much difficulty, but clearly preferred the sweet fruit purees over the vegetables. The problems started at 10 months of age, when Robert was introduced to stage 3 baby food, which caused a lot of gagging. Mrs. Camp decided to skip the stage 3 baby food and advanced him to table food. Robert enjoyed feeding himself some dry cereal but did not like to feed himself with the spoon, wanted his mother to feed him the yogurt, and put out his hands to be wiped if they got "messy." As he was introduced to beans and peas, he experienced severe gagging and consequently refused to open his mouth and cried if his mother continued offering them to him. The same happened with the introduction of eggs and soft chicken meat. After several episodes of gagging, Robert became very vigilant about what foods his mother offered him and refused to be fed by her except for the pureed baby foods and yogurt. He learned to feed himself and became very selective about which foods he would accept. This way, he eliminated all vegetables, most fruits, meats, and eggs, and he could never be persuaded to try pizza.

Additional Hypersensitivities

In addition to their Sensory Food Aversions, many of these children experience hypersensitivities in other sensory areas as well (Smith, Roux, Naidoo, & Venter, 2005). Parents frequently report that these children do not like to get their hands "messy," do not like to have their teeth brushed or their hair washed, become distressed when asked to walk on grass or sand, or to wear socks or shoes, certain fabrics, or labels on clothing. Many of these children are also hypersensitive to smells, and some may have difficulty with loud sounds and bright lights.

The following case describes a young child who in addition to his Sensory Food Aversions showed symptoms of hypersensitivity to touch of certain textures and to sounds:

Example: Joshua was 3 years old when he was referred for an evaluation because of his limited diet and his refusal to eat most nutritious foods. He ate the same foods every day for breakfast, lunch, and dinner. The foods he ate included dry Cheerios, yogurt, pudding, an occasional waffle or pancake, and a wide variety of snack items, including chips, crackers, cookies, fruit snacks, candies, and ice cream. He did not eat any meat, poultry, fish, vegetables, fruit, pasta, cheese, eggs, bread, potatoes, or pizza. He drank a formula, enriched with calories, vitamins, and minerals, and he liked fruit juice.

Joshua's birth history was unremarkable. He was breast-fed for 4 weeks, but he was a very slow feeder, and his mother decided to switch him to bottle feedings. When switched to bottle feedings, initially he had some difficulty with the nipple but did well with an orthodontic nipple. At 4 months, he was introduced to baby food. He did well with cereal, fruits, and orange vegetables, but refused all meats and other vegetables. He would gag or vomit when his parents tried to advance him to the stage 3 combination foods, or if he got an undesired food into his mouth. He was started on table foods around 10 to 12 months and initially did well with pureed items. When offered solid foods, he would touch them to his tongue and then refuse them. However, he had no difficulty eating a wide variety of snack items and quickly learned to differentiate what foods he liked from those he did not want, and he refused to open his mouth if he did not want to eat the food.

In regard to Joshua's sensory profile, he became extremely upset if his hands, face, or clothing got messy. He wanted his hands or face washed immediately and wanted the item of clothing off his body. He did not start feeding himself with utensils until he was almost 3 years old, and he became very fearful that there might be spilling of food and he might get messy. He could not tolerate if foods would mix on his plate, and he would use a different spoon for each food item. He did not like walking or sitting on grass, but did not have any difficulty walking or playing in sand at the beach. He was also very sensitive to certain noises, especially if they were loud. He would awaken at night in response to the garbage truck or a snow plow coming down his street, and he would be frightened by these sounds.

Course and Natural History

The prevalence study by Carruth and colleagues (2004) demonstrated that there is a steady increase in picky eaters between 4 and 24 months of age. As the case histories described above illustrate, some of the children with Sensory Food Aversions become already symptomatic in the first few weeks of life, or they may have difficulties with the introduction of baby foods, but most children do not limit their food choices and refuse to try any new foods until the toddler years. A longitudinal study of children's food preferences by Skinner, Carruth, Bounds, and Ziegler (2002), who followed children from 2–3 years to 8 years of age, found that the number of foods liked at 8 years was predicted by the number liked at 4 years of age. Children were more likely to accept newly tasted foods between 2 and 4 years of age than during school age. These studies and my clinical observation indicate that the toddler years are critical in the development of food preferences.

If children have aversive reactions to food during this developmental period, the way the parents handle their distress and manage their food refusal seems to play an important role in whether the children can overcome the fear of trying other foods that remind them of the aversive food. Children who remain fearful will avoid any food that appears to evoke "feeling memories" of aversive experiences they had in the past. Most older children with Sensory Food Aversions cannot explain why they refuse to eat foods that they have never tried. They will say, "I know that the food will taste badly or feel badly in my mouth," and they are puzzled by their own inability to explain themselves any better. Given that most children have their aversive experiences as infants or toddlers, when they are cognitively not mature enough to verbally link cause and effect, they seem to be left only with feeling memories triggered by looking at a new food that they associate with a food that caused aversive reactions when they were younger. Few older children can shed light on their fear of trying certain foods. One precocious 7-year-old explained to me why he did not want to eat any yellow foods. His mother said that he was already talking in sentences at the age of 1, and he explained to me that when he was little (which was at 18 months of age), his mother gave him yellow squash, which made him vomit, and now he was afraid that other yellow foods would do the same thing. Another 11-year-old expressed to me that he was afraid to eat any meat because when he was 5 years old, his mother gave him chicken, which made him vomit, and "it messed up his brain."

Most preschool children with Sensory Food Aversions are very fixed on what foods they will eat, and they usually react very strongly and become distressed if the adults try to make them eat a food they do not want. One of my little patients came home crying from pre-school and refused to go back the next day. With much patience, his parents were finally able to get him to open up and to tell them that the teacher had said that he had to eat the snack food that all the other children were eating. He told his parents that he was scared, and that he could not eat the food, and that's why he started crying. The same little boy did not want to sit at the table with the rest of the family during dinner time because he did not like the smell of their food, and he did not want to look at their food.

However, there are some preschoolers who may refuse to try any new foods at home but, when watching their peers enjoying their food, become encouraged to try the food themselves (Birch, Zimmerman, & Hind, 1980). In general, as indicated in the study by Skinner and colleagues (2002), children between the ages of 4 and 7 or 8 years are very set in their food preferences. When children are around 7 to 8 years old, they seem to become more socially aware of their peers, and some become self-conscious that they are afraid to eat the foods their peers seem to enjoy. They may become embarrassed when they are at their friend's house and are afraid to eat any of the foods that are offered. They may avoid social functions that include meals, such as sleepovers and birthday parties, and when they get older, they may be afraid to go to summer camp. Some of these children continue to engage in struggles over food with their parents because of their limited diet, which often consists of sweet and salty snack foods and no vegetables, fruits, or meats. Mealtimes can cause immense anxiety not only for the child but for other family members as well and lead to frequent mealtime battles. Some parents resign themselves to the limited diet of their children, and they give them vitamin supplements or enriched breakfast drinks. They try to find restaurants where they can order something the child eats, and they pack special foods for the child when they travel.

For some children, the fear of trying new foods and the social limitations may lead to general anxiety, obsessive compulsive symptoms, and school difficulties (Timimi et al., 1997). On the other hand, some parents of children with Sensory Food Aversions report that they themselves were unable to eat a variety of foods as young children but learned to eat new foods primarily during their adolescent or young adult years, when they wanted to fit in with their peers.

Etiology

There are no empirical studies that have examined the etiology of Sensory Food Aversions in infants and toddlers. However, research with preschool and older children and with adults has related taste sensitivities to the bitter substances PROP (propylthiouracil) and PTC (phenylthiocarbamide) to strong food preferences and to the number of fungiform papillae and taste buds on the individual's tongue (Duffy & Bartoshuck, 2000). There is growing evidence suggesting that there are three groups of tasters: supertasters, medium tasters, and nontasters who perceive the bitterness of PROP as very to intensely strong, moderate to strong, or weak, respectively. The genetic locus influencing sensitivity to PROP has been characterized by Reed and colleagues (1999), and the gene that determines PTC sensitivity has been identified by Kim and colleagues (2003). It has been suggested that supertaster status requires both a high density of fungiform papillae and taste buds and two dominant alleles of the PROP gene (Bartoshuk et al., 2001). Compared to nontasters, supertasters experience greater subjective burn and irritation from pepperlike substances, greater fattiness of fat-containing foods, and greater dislikes of foods with a high fat content. Studies by Miller and Reedy (1990) and by Essick, Chopra, Guest, and McGlone (2003) revealed that the fungiform papillae on the tip of the tongue of the three taster groups differed in both density and diameter, and the diameter decreased linearly with density, with the supertasters having the greatest density of fungiform papillae. These authors found that individuals who differ in the extent to which they perceive bitterness to PROP also differ in lingual tactile acuity. Individuals who rated bitterness in PROP as very strong (supertasters) were found to be twice as tactually acute in identifying different letters of the alphabet put on the tongue than nontasters. Therefore, it is likely that supertasters will not only appreciate bitter tastes but also detect more readily small particles and granularity in food and be more sensitive to food grit and contaminants. This finding has helped me to understand when older children with Sensory Food Aversions describe that both the taste and the texture of the food are bothering them.

In addition to these genetic studies pointing to the heritability of taste and texture sensitivity, some studies have examined the heritability of food neophobia, the fear of trying new foods, which is one of the characteristics of Sensory Food Aversions. A study by Cooke, Haworth, and Wardle (2007), which examined food neophobia in a large sample of twins age 8–11 years, estimated that 78% was heritable and 22% of the variance was explained by nonshared environmental factors. A study of the heritability of food neophobia by Knaapila and colleagues (2007) examined Finnish families and British twins, and yielded similar results. Knaapila et al. concluded that in both populations about two thirds of the variation in food neophobia was genetically determined. In addition, Galloway, Lee, and Birch (2003) found that food neophobia in 7-year-old girls was predicted by traitlike variables: their mothers' high food neophobia and their own high levels of anxiety. This latter finding of high anxiety in these children with food neophobia agrees with my clinical experience that children with Sensory Food Aversions tend to be prone to anxiety, which may show up in other areas as well. Young children may demonstrate more severe separation anxiety, and older children may develop school phobia, social phobia, or obsessive-compulsive symptoms such as frequent hand washing. An adolescent boy with Sensory Food Aversions described to me that when he sat in front of a hamburger (a new food he was trying to conquer), he felt his heart racing and his hands getting sweaty, and he started feeling nauseous. He had to stop trying to eat the hamburger and get up and do something else before he was able to recover from his anxiety.

Although the above studies indicate a high heritability of taste and texture sensitivities, as well as of the fear of trying new foods, they do not explain the whole picture of Sensory Food Aversions. Leann Birch (1999) pointed out that several factors contribute to the development of food preferences. She postulated that whether genetic predispositions are manifested in food preferences that foster healthy diets depends on the eating environment, including food availability and the child-feeding practices of the adults. This begins with breast-feeding versus formula. A study by Sullivan and Birch (1994) of 4- to 6-month-old infants demonstrated that after 10 opportunities to consume vegetables, all infants significantly increased their intake. Although the infants did not differ initially, infants fed breast milk showed greater increases in vegetable intake after exposure and had an overall greater level of intake than formula-fed infants. It has been known that the diet of rat pups is influenced by maternal diet during lactation (Galef & Henderson, 1972) and that the sensory qualities of human milk are influenced by the mother's diet and result in changes that can be detected by the infant. However, the infants and their mothers in the study by Sullivan and Birch were not screened for picky eating or food neophobia. Consequently, it is not clear why some infants were breast-fed and others were fed formula, what kind of diet the mothers were eating themselves, and whether any of these infants had a genetic predisposition for Sensory Food Aversions. Birch and Marlin (1982) also reported that 5–10 exposures of a new food were necessary for 2-year-olds to see an increased preference for it. Although repeated opportunities to taste a new food reduced food neophobia and enhanced acceptance, repeated opportunities to smell or look at the food did not.

However, the way parents present foods plays an important role in children's acceptance (Fisher & Birch, 1999). When children are given certain foods as rewards for approved behaviors, enhanced preference of those foods results (Birch, Marlin, & Rotter, 1984). However, when children are offered rewards for eating (e.g., "if you eat your vegetables, you can watch TV"), the foods eaten to obtain rewards become less preferred (Newman & Taylor, 1992).

It has long been known that humans associate foods' flavors with the consequences that follow eating. These consequences can be positive, and repeated associations of food sensory cues with positive posteating experiences can lead to learned preferences. On the other hand, Schafe and Bernstein (1996) described how negative gastrointestinal consequences of nausea and emesis lead to learned aversion. Once an aversion has been formed, the food will be avoided, and a single aversive experience can lead to avoidance of that food for decades (Garb & Stunkard, 1974; Logue, Ophir, & Strauss, 1981; Schafe & Bernstein, 1996). Mattes (1991) noted family resemblances in food aversions formation, with some families more prone to learned food aversions than others. He also reported that aversions were formed most readily to protein foods of animal origin: Aversions to eggs, meats, and seafood were most common. In her review of the development of food preferences, Birch (1999) raises the question of whether children with chronic feeding problems, who are described as fussy or finicky eaters, may have restricted diets as a result of multiple learned food aversions.

Integrating the findings from the studies described above with my clinical experience, I have developed a gene–environment interaction model to understand Sensory Food Aversions. According to this model, children who have inherited sensitivities to the taste, texture, temperature, or smell of certain foods may experience aversive reactions when ingesting these foods. These reactions may be mild, as indicated by the child's grimacing, or more severe and result in spitting out the food, gagging, and vomiting. If the child has also inherited a vulnerability to become fearful (as indicated by the genetic studies on food neophobia), the child will associate the aversive food with the experience of having to spit it out, with gagging or vomiting, and the child will become afraid to eat the food again. Fearful children will also generalize from the aversive reaction to one food to other foods that look similar in color or appearance and will consequently refuse to eat whole food groups. They will be afraid to try any new foods out of fear that the new food may cause them to have an aversive reaction.

This feeding disorder can become symptomatic in the first year of life, and amazingly, very young infants already have the ability to learn by association, as indicated by their behavior. They will refuse to drink from the bottle if the content of the bottle is aversive to them, but they may accept food from the spoon or vice versa. If parents do not understand the infant's or child's food refusal and try hard to get their child to accept the foods by coaxing, bargaining, threatening, or force-feeding, the child will become more and more fearful and increasingly restrictive in his acceptance of foods. Parents and children become trapped in struggles for control, all feeling helpless and frustrated.

Treatment

Because no empirical studies have systematically examined how to best treat infants and young children with Sensory Food Aversions, through clinical experience, I have learned that parents are better able to follow suggestions for how to deal with their child when they have an increased understanding of their child's problems. Therefore, I usually start the intervention by exploring the parents' own feeding and eating histories to relate the child's difficulty with the texture, taste, temperature, or smell of certain foods to difficulties one or the other parent may have had as a child. Then I outline the gene–environment model described above, to help the parents understand that their child has probably more taste buds and more sensory receptors for taste, texture, and smell, which give the child a more intense experience of some qualities of certain foods, and this heightened sensitivity makes these foods aversive. After this groundwork has been done, I give specific recommendations on how the parents may best help their child.

If infants or toddlers show strong aversive reactions to a new food–such as spitting the food out, gagging, or vomiting–the parents are best advised to give up on having the child eat this food. Repeated exposure to aversive foods tends to increase the infant's or young child's fearfulness and food refusal. On the other hand, if the infant just grimaces, the parents may expose the infant to the new food at another time and pair a small amount of the aversive food with a preferred food. A gradual increase of the aversive food over several meals may allow the infant to get used to the new food.

For toddlers, modeling the eating of new foods by the parents and waiting until the toddler asks to try the food generally is more effective than putting new foods on the toddler's plate and asking the toddler to try them. There is nothing more challenging for a toddler than not to be offered a food that the parents seem to enjoy. The harder the parents make it for the toddler to get hold of their food, the more the toddler wants it. I advise parents that if the toddler wants their food, they should say, "This is Mommy's or Daddy's food, but I will give you a little piece." Usually, the toddler is so keen to get the food that he or she is less focused on the taste or texture of the food. If the parents stay neutral as to whether the toddler likes the requested food or not, the toddler will remain neutral as well and decide whether he or she likes the food. If a food of the parents is aversive to the toddler, the toddler will spit it out and not want to eat it again, but he or she will not be scared to ask for another food from their plate. On the other hand, if parents put food on the toddler's plate and ask the toddler to try it, the toddler may be very tempted to refuse it. Children in general and toddlers in particular are more willing to try new foods if it is in their control.

Once children fear trying new foods, their diet becomes more and more limited, and by 3 to 4 years old, many children are no longer swayed by what their parents eat. Occasionally, young children may be willing to try new foods in a preschool setting, but more often they become anxious in social situations and try to avoid eating with others. Preschool children who have limited their diet and have become fearful of trying new foods are of a particular treatment challenge. The best some parents can do to help these children is to continue eating a variety of foods without offering them to the child and to accommodate the child by always preparing foods that the child can eat without fear. It is best to avoid any conflict by making the child's limited diet a nonissue. Because some of these children may eat only a handful of foods and tend to get tired of a food after a while if they eat it every day, it is advisable to rotate the foods from one meal to another or from day to day.

These recommendations can be very hard on parents, particularly if the child's diet is limited and deficient in essential micronutrients. Consequently, it is important to analyze the child's food intake and to supplement the missing nutrients. There are formulas for infants that contain all the important nutrients, and there are pediatric formulas for toddlers and children that provide the essential nutrients for growth. Sometimes it is difficult to find a formula that the child will accept, and the parents may have to offer different flavors or different types of formula until the child is able to drink it. For children who are primarily avoiding vegetables and fruits but are drinking milk, supplementation with vitamins may be adequate. In any case, a thorough nutritional assessment of the child's diet is necessary to determine which nutrients may have to be supplemented. The supplements provide a safety net for the child's growth and allow the parents to neutralize the conflict over eating within the family.

Once this groundwork has been laid, the parents need help with how to manage mealtime within the family and how to help their child develop internal regulation of eating in spite of his difficulties with certain foods. The parents are introduced to the feeding guidelines described in detail in the previous chapter on Infantile Anorexia. Because children with Sensory Food Aversions often get anxious and restless during mealtime, they need to learn to sit at the table and relax. This often requires taking a time-out for self-calming, which is also described in the previous chapter on Infantile Anorexia. Many children with Sensory Food Aversions also show a strong preference for sweet snack foods and candy, and the parents are advised to neutralize the "sweetness" of these foods by making small amounts of these foods part of the meal, but not to offer them with every meal, and to allow the child to eat the candy first if the child wants it that way. However, there should be no candy or sweet snack food outside of scheduled meal and snack times. Parents are often surprised that their young children lose interest in the sweet foods once they are not "special" anymore and are not associated with being a "treat." One mother who had two little girls, one with serious feeding difficulties, was worried that the children were asking her all day long about wanting M&M's. I advised her to put a few M&M's on the children's plate along with the rest of the food. To the mother's surprise, after only 3 days, the children forgot their M&M's and left them on the plate.

Because some of the toddlers with Sensory Food Aversions avoid any foods that require significant chewing, such as hard vegetables or meats, they may become delayed in oral motor and expressive speech development. These children can benefit from oral motor and speech therapy.

Once mealtime conflict has been eliminated, some children begin to relax and may even ask to try a new food that they see their parents or siblings eat. However, others stay with their limited diet and take supplements to compensate for their dietary deficiencies. Some of the children whom I had seen as preschoolers returned for treatment when they were 7 to 10 years old and wanted to work on overcoming their fear of trying new foods. These older children established a hierarchy of foods that they wanted to learn to eat. In this hierarchy, each food is assigned a number indicating how scary it is to eat, with 10 being the *most scary* and 1 being the *least scary*. Then the children start with the least scary food and are given "a point for courage" for each bite of the new food they eat. They are rewarded for the first 10 points and the final 50 points for the new food they learn to eat. I have learned that once they have eaten 50 bites of a new food, they are usually able to incorporate the food into their diet, and they start with the next food. The parents serve as "coaches" by buying or preparing the food and assisting the child when he or she tries the food. However, the child is determining how many bites at any trial he or she wants to eat. At the beginning, the children are often eating only one or two bites at any one time, and they often struggle with the taste and texture of the new food until they have had 15 to 25 bites. Occasionally, they are surprised that the new food tastes quite good, and at other times, they find that it takes more than 50 bites until they are really comfortable with the new food. In general, the desensitization to new foods is slow, but the children continue with encouragement, and gradually they conquer one food after the other.

The following case illustrates the development of symptoms, the assessment by our Multidisciplinary Feeding Disorders Team, and the treatment of a toddler with Sensory Food Aversions.

Example: Cathy was 2½ years old when she was brought for an assessment by the Multidisciplinary Feeding Disorders Team because she refused to eat vegetables, fruits, and meats. Her parents had started to give her a multivitamin daily, but they were worried that she was missing other essential nutrients in her limited diet, and they were concerned that her articulation was so poor that nobody outside of the family could understand what she was saying. Her daily diet consisted of Cheerios or pancakes in the morning, peanut butter sandwiches, some cheese (which had to be American), pasta, cake, crackers, ice cream, and milk during the rest of the day.

Her feeding problems started when she was introduced to baby food. She accepted baby food sweetened with fruit but grimaced when given baby food with vegetables and spat it out. She gagged when introduced to baby food with lumps of meat, and she refused to accept any baby food after that. At 9 months of age, Cathy was offered soft table foods, which she ate only if she could finger-feed herself. She had another episode of gagging when introduced to green beans at 15 months of age, and consequently refused to touch any green vegetables and fruits. She never tried any meats, and she became very distressed when her parents, Mr. and Mrs. Long, put any food on her plate that she did not want. When her parents insisted that she should at least try one bite of a new food before she could leave the table, Cathy cried throughout the whole meal and ate nothing, not even her preferred foods. Mr. and Mrs. Long had strong disagreements about how to handle Cathy's food refusal. Mr. Long had similar food dislikes as a child and wanted to leave her alone. Mrs. Long was very concerned about Cathy's health because of her limited diet, and she tried bribing, coaxing, distracting, and threatening just to get Cathy to try new foods. Both parents experienced mealtime as very stressful and felt that Cathy was getting increasingly rigid about her food likes and dislikes.

The observation of feeding revealed intense conflict between Cathy and Mrs. Long regarding the various foods she refused to eat. Cathy ate well as long as her mother offered her preferred foods, but cried and pushed the food away if she did not want it. The observation of free play showed an engaging give-and-take relationship between Cathy and her parents.

The nutritional assessment showed that Cathy was growing at the 30th percentile for height and the 25th percentile for weight, with a head circumference at the 30th percentile. Although Cathy was taking in adequate calories, she was not getting enough zinc and iron from her diet, and without the multivitamin, her diet was deficient in several vitamins.

The oral motor assessment revealed that Cathy used an immature chewing pattern that was felt to be due to her lack of practice with chewing crunchy and chewy foods. This oral motor delay was felt to account for her articulation problems.

The nutritionist on the team recommended that the parents obtain vitamins complete with zinc and iron in order to compensate for the nutrients missing in Cathy's diet. The occupational therapist felt that there were no limitations to Cathy's oral motor movements and with practice Cathy would develop a more mature chewing pattern. However, she suggested that Cathy receive speech therapy to help with her articulation problems. The gastroenterologist felt that Cathy was growing at a normal rate and that her overall health was good. The psychiatrist explained to Mr. and Mrs. Long the diagnosis of Sensory Food Aversions and invited the parents to come back for more suggestions on how to handle Cathy's food refusal and the family meals.

It was suggested to Mr. and Mrs. Long that they offer Cathy only the foods that she had been accepting willingly in the past, which meant that Mrs. Long had to prepare separate meals for her. Mrs. Long could ask Cathy what she wanted to eat, but once Cathy had made her choice, that was what Mrs. Long would offer. If Cathy was going to be difficult and not decide what she wanted, Mrs. Long would decide for her among the foods Cathy had eaten in the past. Once Mrs. Long had prepared the food and put it on the table, there were no other choices to be made by Cathy. The parents were to eat their regular meals without offering any of their foods to Cathy. If Cathy were to ask for any of their food, they were to give her only a small piece of their food and say, "This is Mommy's food, but I'll give you a little piece." They were not to praise her if she liked the food nor become disappointed if she did not want to have it anymore.

The feeding guidelines (described in the chapter on Infantile Anorexia) were then discussed with Mr. and Mrs. Long. The parents had no difficulty agreeing on a regular meal and afternoon snack schedule, but they anticipated problems with Cathy asking for candy and ice cream when they went out to the mall or when she just wanted a treat. It was suggested that they offer ice cream and candy on some days and let Cathy decide whether she wanted to eat it first or later in the meal, but if she asked for sweets outside of mealtime, they should tell her, "We will have some during one of our next meals." The parents also anticipated problems with keeping Cathy at the table until they were finished with the meal. The therapist went over the time-out procedure (also described in the chapter on Infantile Anorexia) and suggested that they explain to Cathy that she was expected to sit at the table until "Mommy's and Daddy's tummies were full" and if she continued to get up, that she would be given only one warning and then put in time-out. It was very important that, after she had completed her time-out, she had to return to the table and the parents were to sit with her and eat for at least 5 minutes to help her understand what they expected from her.

After 3 weeks, Mr. and Mrs. Long came back for another session to discuss how Cathy had responded to the suggested changes. They reported that when asked what she wanted to eat, Cathy had asked for foods that she then refused, and Mrs. Long had decided not to ask her anymore and just make the choices for Cathy. This had made mealtimes much easier, and there was no more conflict about what Cathy was eating. They had not offered her any of their foods, and Cathy had not asked to try any of the parents' food. As predicted, Cathy had a very difficult time staying in her seat and had received her first time-out for getting up and running around. However, she learned quickly and accepted that she had to wait until "Mommy's and Daddy's tummies were full." They were surprised that she had stopped asking for candy since they put some on her plate at some meals, but she had more difficulty with not getting ice cream when they went to the mall. Overall, the parents felt very relieved that they had gotten back some order in their lives and that mealtimes were not so stressful anymore. Mr. and Mrs. Long were reminded that in case Cathy were to ask for one of the foods that they were eating, they should give her a small piece only, to stay neutral whether she liked it or not, and to give her more only if she asked for more.

When last seen, Mr. and Mrs. Long reported that Cathy had made nice progress with the help of speech therapy, and at the age of 3 years was articulating well. After having stopped offering Cathy any new food for about 2 months, Cathy surprised her mother by asking her to have some of her peach. She liked it and asked for more on another day. Gradually, she began to eat soft fruits without the peel, and after several months, she tried chicken nuggets. Her diet increased in variety very slowly, and when she entered preschool at the age of 3, she tried a number of foods at school that she had not touched at home. Her diet became more complete. However, at the age of 4, Cathy was still not able to eat the variety of foods the rest of her family enjoyed.

Differential Diagnosis and Comorbidity

As I discussed in the chapter on Infantile Anorexia, both Sensory Food Aversions and Infantile Anorexia primarily present in the pure form but can also occur with one another. Although children with pure Sensory Food Aversions usually have a good appetite if they are given their preferred foods, children with comorbid Sensory Food Aversions and Infantile Anorexia may not only be selective about what foods they are willing to accept but also eat very little. These children can become underweight because they also have poor awareness of their hunger feelings, which is the hallmark of Infantile Anorexia. When presented with these cases, it is very important to diagnose and treat both feeding disorders, which I will explain in more detail in the chapter on Comorbidities and Complex Feeding Disorders.

Some infants or toddlers become so afraid to eat after they have had aversive experiences, such as severe gagging or vomiting, or after they have been force-fed an aversive food, that they develop a Posttraumatic Feeding Disorder, which I describe in chapter 6.

As I have explained in this chapter, food neophobia (the fear of eating new foods) is part of the problem in Sensory Food Aversions, and many of the children become very anxious around mealtimes. Some children show anxiety in other areas, which may manifest as separation anxiety in young children and as school phobia or social phobia in school-age children. Other children may have fears of bugs or dogs, and some develop obsessive–compulsive symptoms such as washing their hands frequently, lining up objects in a certain order, or getting very upset if what they are doing is not perfect. These anxiety disorders are often related to intense family conflict around eating, and consequently it is important to neutralize the family conflict at mealtime and to address the child's anxiety if it does not respond to the interventions described above.

References

Bartoshuk, L. M., Duffy, V. B., Fast, K., Kveton, J. F., Lucchina, L. A., Phillips, M. N., et al. (2001). What makes a supertaster? [Abstract]. *Chemical Senses, 26,* 1074.

Birch, L. L. (1999). Development of food preferences. *Annual Review of Nutrition, 19,* 41–62.

Birch, L. L., & Marlin, D. W. (1982). I don't like it; I never tried it: Effects of exposure to food on two-year-old children's food preferences. *Appetite, 4,* 353–360.

Birch, L. L., Marlin, D. W., & Rotter, J. (1984). Eating as the "means" activity in a contingency: Effect on young children's food preference. *Child Development, 55,* 432–439.

Birch, L. L., Zimmerman, S., & Hind, H. (1980). The influence of social-affective context on preschool children's food preferences. *Child Development, 51,* 856–861.

Carruth, B. R., Ziegler, P. J., Gordon, A., & Barr, S. I. (2004). Prevalence of picky eaters among infants and toddlers and their caregivers' decisions about offering a new food. *Journal of the American Dietetic Association, 104*(Suppl. 1), S57–S64.

Chatoor, I., & Ammaniti, M. (2007). A classification of feeding disorders of infancy and early childhood. In W. E. Narrow, M. B. First, P. Sirovatka, & D. A. Regier (Eds.), *Age and gender considerations in psychiatric diagnosis: A research agenda for DSM-V* (pp. 227–242). Arlington, VA: American Psychiatric Press.

Cooke, L. J., Haworth, C. M., & Wardle, J. (2007). Genetic and environmental influences on children's food neophobia. *The American Journal of Clinical Nutrition, 86,* 428–433.

Dovey, T. M., Staples, P. A., Gibson, E. L., & Halford, J. C. (2007). Food neophobia and 'picky/fussy' eating: A review. *Appetite, 50*(2-3), 181–193.

Duffy, V. B, & Bartoshuk, L. M. (2000). Food acceptance and genetic variation in taste. *Journal of the American Dietetic Association, 100,* 647–655.

Essick, G. K., Chopra, A., Guest, S., & McGlone, F. (2003). Lingual tactile acuity, taste perception, and the density and diameter of fungiform papillae in female subjects. *Physiology & Behavior, 80,* 289–302.

Fisher, J. O., & Birch, L. L. (1999). Restricting access to a palatable food affects children's behavioral response, food selection, and intake. *The American Journal of Clinical Nutrition, 69,* 1264–1272.

Galef, B. G., & Henderson, P. W. (1972). Mother's milk: A determinant of the feeding preferences of weaning rat pups. *Journal of Comparative and Physiological Psychology, 78*(2), 213–219.

Galloway, A. T., Lee, Y., & Birch, L. L. (2003). Predictors and consequences of food neophobia and pickiness in young girls. *Journal of the American Dietetic Association, 103,* 692–698.

Garb, J. L., & Stunkard, A. J. (1974). Taste aversions in man. *The American Journal of Psychiatry, 131,* 1204–1207.

Jacobi, C., Agras, W. S., Bryson, S., & Hammer, L. D. (2003). Behavioral validation, precursors, and concomitants of picky eating in childhood. *Journal of the American Academy of Child and Adolescent Psychiatry, 42*(1), 76–84.

Kim, U., Jorgenson, E., Coon, H., Leppert, M., Risch, N., & Drayna, D. (2003). Positional cloning of the human quantitative trait locus underlying taste sensitivity to phenylthiocarbamide. *Science, 299,* 1221–1225.

Knaapila, A., Tuorila, H., Silventoinen, K., Keskitalo, K., Kallela, M., Wessman, M., et al. (2007). Food neophobia shows heritable variation in humans. *Physiology & Behavior, 91*, 573–578.

Logue, A. W., Ophir, I., & Strauss, K. (1981). The acquisition of taste aversions in humans. *Behaviour Research and Therapy, 19*, 319–333.

Marchi, M., & Cohen, P. (1990). Early childhood eating behaviors and adolescent eating disorders. *Journal of the American Academy of Child and Adolescent Psychiatry, 29*, 112–117.

Mattes, R. D. (1991). Learned food aversions: A family study. *Physiology and Behavior, 50*, 499–504.

Miller, I. J., & Reedy, F. E. (1990). Variations in human taste bud density and taste intensity perception. *Physiology & Behavior, 47*, 1213–1219.

Narrow, W. E., First, M. B., Sirovatka, P., & Regier, D. A. (Eds.). (2007). *Age and gender considerations in psychiatric diagnosis: A research agenda for DSM-V*. Arlington, VA: American Psychiatric Press.

Newman, J., & Taylor, A. (1992). Effect of a means-end contingency on young children's food preferences. *Journal of Experimental Child Psychology, 53*(2), 200–216.

Reed, D. R., Nanthakumar, E., North, M., Bell, C., Bartoshuk, L. M., & Price, R. A. (1999). Localization of a gene for bitter taste perception to human chromosome 5p15. *The American Journal of Human Genetics, 64*, 1478–1480.

Rydell, A. M., Dahl, M., & Sundelin, C. (1995). Characteristics of school children who are choosy eaters. *The Journal of Genetic Psychology, 156*(2), 217–229.

Schafe, G. E., & Bernstein, I. L. (1996). Taste aversion learning. In E. D. Capaldi (Ed.), *Why we eat what we eat: The psychology of eating* (pp. 31–51). Washington, DC: American Psychological Association.

Skinner, J. D., Carruth, B. R., Bounds, W., & Ziegler, P. J. (2002). Children's food preferences: A longitudinal analysis. *Journal of the American Dietetic Association 102*, 1638–1647.

Smith, A. M., Roux, S., Naidoo, N. T., & Venter, D. J. (2005). Food choices of tactile defensive children. *Nutrition, 21*(1), 14–19.

Sullivan, S. A., & Birch, L. L. (1994). Infant dietary experience and acceptance of solid foods. *Pediatrics, 93*(2), 271–277.

Timimi, S., Douglas, J., & Tsiftsopoulou, K. (1997). Selective eaters: A retrospective case note study. *Child: Care, Health, and Development, 23*(3), 265–278.

ZERO TO THREE. (2005). *Diagnostic classification of mental health and developmental disorders of infancy and early childhood: Revised edition (DC:0–3R)*. Washington, DC: Author.

POSTTRAUMATIC FEEDING DISORDER

Nosology

MY COLLEAGUES and I first described Posttraumatic Eating Disorder in latency-age children in an article in 1988 (Chatoor, Conley, & Dickson). These children refused to eat any solid food after they had experienced an episode of choking or severe gagging. They were preoccupied with the fear of choking and dying. When approached with food, they demonstrated intense anticipatory anxiety and sometimes panic until the food was removed. Later, I (Chatoor, 1991) described this disorder in infants and toddlers as Posttraumatic Feeding Disorder. Parents of these children may report that the infant had one or more episodes of vomiting while having the bottle and consequently started to cry at the sight of the bottle and refused to drink from it anymore. Some parents may report that the infant's refusal to eat any solid food started after an incident of choking or severe gagging. Some parents may have observed that the food refusal followed intubation, the insertion of nasogastric tubes, or major surgery requiring vigorous suctioning (Chatoor, Ganiban, Harrison, & Hirsch, 2001). In all of these cases, the food refusal seemed to follow a traumatic experience to the oropharynx or gastrointestinal tract and seemed to be triggered by intense fear in anticipation of feeding.

Several other clinicians have reported that children and adults can develop a fear of swallowing food after choking and have described it as choking phobia (McNally, 1994; Solyom & Sookman, 1980). A recent review by de Lucas-Taracena and Montañés-Rada (2006) of 41 case reports described that swallowing phobia is characterized by fear of suffocating on swallowing food, drinks, or pills, and that the disorder has been reported in individuals ranging in age from 8 to 78 years. They also report that this disorder has a high comorbidity with anxiety disorders. Some authors use the term *globus hystericus* (Liebowitz, 1987), and still others call it functional dysphagia (Kaplan & Evans, 1978). Although some of these case reports include children, less attention has been paid to this disorder in infants and toddlers. However, Dellert, Hyams, Treem, and Geertsma (1993) reported that 5% of infants with gastroesophageal reflux developed "feeding resistance" to oral feedings severe enough to require tube feedings for nutritional support. Feeding resistance is the central symptom of a Posttraumatic Feeding Disorder, and my colleagues and I (Chatoor et al., 2001) found that toddlers with a Posttraumatic Feeding Disorder could be differentiated from healthy toddlers and from toddlers diagnosed with Infantile Anorexia by the most intense resistance to accepting and swallowing food.

The diagnostic criteria for Posttraumatic Feeding Disorder underwent some changes when I worked with the national Task Force for Research Diagnostic Criteria for Infants and Preschool Children (Scheeringa et al., 2003). The diagnostic criteria for Posttraumatic Feeding Disorder were also published in the *Diagnostic Classification of Mental Health and Developmental Disorders of Infancy and Early Childhood: Revised Edition (DC:0–3R*; ZERO TO THREE, 2005). However, the disorder was named "Feeding Disorder Associated with Insults to the Gastrointestinal Tract." The diagnostic criteria were reviewed and further modified when I worked with the national Infant and Young Child Research Planning Work Group, which was supported by the American Psychiatric Association. These revised criteria for Posttraumatic Feeding Disorder and for five other feeding disorders presented in this book are described in Chatoor and Ammaniti's (2007) chapter in *Age and Gender Considerations in Psychiatric Diagnosis: A Research Agenda for DSM-V* (Narrow, First, Sirovatka, & Regier, 2007). The most recent diagnostic criteria for Posttraumatic Feeding Disorder are presented below.

Diagnostic Criteria

A. This feeding disorder is characterized by the acute onset of severe and consistent food refusal.

B. The onset of the food refusal can occur at any age, from infancy to adulthood.

C. The food refusal follows a traumatic event or repeated traumatic insults to the oropharynx or gastrointestinal tract (e.g., choking, gagging, vomiting, gastroesophageal reflux, insertion of nasogastric or endotracheal tubes, suctioning, force-feeding) that trigger intense distress in the child.

D. Consistent refusal to eat manifests in one of the following ways, depending on the mode of feeding experienced by the child in association with the traumatic event(s), either bottle feeding or feeding of solid food:

- Refuses to drink from the bottle but may accept food offered by spoon. (Although consistently refuses to drink from the bottle when awake, may drink from the bottle when sleepy or asleep.)

- Refuses solid food but may accept the bottle, fluids, or pureed food.

- Refuses all oral feedings.

E. Reminders of the traumatic event(s) cause distress as manifested by one or more of the following:

- Shows anticipatory distress when positioned for feeding.

- Shows intense resistance when approached with bottle or food.

- Shows resistance to swallow food placed in mouth.

F. The food refusal poses an acute and/or long-term threat to the child's health, nutrition, and growth, and threatens the progression of age-appropriate feeding development of the child.

Clinical Presentation

This feeding disorder is characterized by the infant's or toddler's consistent refusal to either drink from the bottle or to eat any solid food, and in severe cases, by the infant's or toddler's refusal to eat at all. Depending on the mode of feeding that the child appears to associate with the traumatic event(s), the child may refuse to eat solids but continue to drink from the bottle, or he may refuse to drink from the bottle but be willing to eat solids (e.g., an infant who choked on a Cheerio refused to eat solids but continued to drink from the bottle, and an infant who experienced vomiting while drinking from the bottle refused the bottle but continued to eat from the spoon).

The onset of the food refusal is frequently rather sudden and follows traumatic experiences that involve the oropharynx or gastrointestinal tract, for example, gagging, choking, vomiting, gastroesophageal reflux, insertion of feeding or endotracheal tubes, or force-feeding. Frequently, the parents are not aware that the event was so frightening to the child that it triggered the food refusal because other children who may undergo the same experience will not necessarily develop a Posttraumatic Feeding Disorder. In my clinical experience, it appears that children who develop a Posttraumatic Feeding Disorder are more prone to anxiety and/or are more sensitive to pain than the average child. Older children who refused to eat solid food after an incident of gagging or choking told me that they were afraid that the food would get stuck in their throat and choke them to death. Infants and young children express this fear through their behavior by crying in anticipation of being fed; when seeing the high chair, the bib, the bottle, or the spoon; or when positioned for feeding. The child cries when approached with food, refuses to open her mouth, arches away from the food, and bats away the bottle or spoon. Some infants or children are brave enough to put the food in their mouth but cannot bring themselves to swallow it (Chatoor et al., 2001). They keep the food in their cheeks and spit it out later. In severe cases, the infants refuse to feed all together. Without supplementation (e.g., intravenous fluids, nasogastric or gastrostomy tube feedings with fortified formula preparations, or parenteral nutrition), some infants and children are in acute danger of dehydration because their fear of eating and drinking appears to override any awareness of hunger or thirst.

Often the food refusal of these children is so intense that it causes severe anxiety in the parents. They may try to coax and distract the child, offer various types of food, and try to feed the child day and night without success. However, some very young infants who are afraid to drink from the bottle when they are awake may drink when they are asleep, not aware of what they are doing. However, if they wake up and see the bottle, they usually push it away and cry.

The following example illustrates the distress of a young infant who refused to drink from the bottle when awake and had started to refuse to accept food from the spoon as well:

Example: Grace was 7 months old when she was referred by a gastroen-terologist for an urgent psychiatric evaluation because of severe crying when offered the bottle and refusal to drink unless she was almost fully asleep and seemed unaware of her feeding.

Mrs. Cook, the mother, reported that Grace was a 7-pound, full-term baby who had a vigorous suck and was feeding well from birth. However, after a few weeks she started to spit up during and after feedings, and by 3 months she developed projectile vomiting. In spite of the frequent vomiting, she gained weight until she was about 4 months of age, when she was referred to a gastroenterologist and diagnosed with gastroe-sophageal reflux. She was given several reflux medications, but she continued to vomit, although less frequently. By 6 months of age, Grace started to arch herself during feedings as if she were in pain. She would cry and refuse to continue with the feeding, but after a break of 5 to 10 minutes, Mrs. Cook was able to coax her into resuming feeding, until she would arch again, cry, and stop feeding altogether. Soon after this behavior started, Mrs. Cook noticed that Grace would start to cry at the sight of the bottle, and she refused to accept the bottle totally as long as she was awake. To stave off starvation, Mrs. Cook relied on feeding her during the night when she was asleep. Grace's food intake greatly diminished, and she started to lose weight. Mrs. Cook tried to introduce solid food, but Grace seemed to have difficulty moving the food in her mouth and spit most of it out.

At the time of referral, Mrs. Cook was exhausted and frightened because of Grace's continued weight loss. A recent gastroscopic examination by the gastroenterologist had shown that the gastroesophageal reflux was markedly improved, that she had only mild redness of the esophagus, and that Grace's ongoing feeding difficulties could not be explained by her medical condition.

The observation of mother and infant during feeding revealed that Grace became distressed the moment her mother positioned her for feeding, and she started to cry and arch herself as soon as she saw the bottle. Her mother put the bottle away and tried to comfort her, but it took more than 10 minutes until Grace could settle in her mother's arms. When Mrs. Cook got the bottle and tried to feed her again, Grace cried even louder and could not be calmed until the bottle was out of her sight. When Mrs. Cook tried to feed her some purees from the spoon, she batted the spoon away and did not want to have anything put in her mouth.

Course and Natural History

For children like Grace, research does not tell us much regarding the course or duration of their Posttraumatic Feeding Disorder. However, individual clinical cases indicate that many infants and children get locked into the fear of eating. Some infants may never accept the bottle, except when they are asleep. They may learn to drink fluids, but not milk, from the cup. They may get their nutrition primarily from purees fed by spoon, and then progress to table food. Some toddlers may drink milk from the bottle and may eat only pureed food until they reach school age, when the social embarrassment of their eating behavior causes the parents to seek help. In severe cases, when the infants refuse all food, gastrostomy feedings have to be implemented, and some children depend on gastrostomy feedings for years.

Etiology

In my observation of infants with a Posttraumatic Feeding Disorder, it appears that their food refusal is caused by fear of eating. They show anticipatory fear when they see reminders of the feeding (e.g., the bottle, bib, or high chair) and become distressed when they are positioned for feeding and when they are approached with food. If any food gets into their mouth, they spit it out or pocket it because they seem afraid to swallow it. These behaviors are very similar to what has been observed in older children and adults who have a Posttraumatic Feeding Disorder (Chatoor et al., 1988) or are described to suffer from choking or swallowing phobia (de Lucas-Taracena & Montañés-Rada, 2006). However, no empirical studies have been done to explain why only some infants with distressing experiences to the oropharynx or gastrointestinal tract develop a Posttraumatic Feeding Disorder. In my clinical observation I found that these children seem very bright and vigilant and appear more prone to react with anxiety than other infants and toddlers who may have similar painful or frightening experiences without becoming fearful afterwards.

Treatment

Because of the complexity of many of these cases, particularly those that result from trauma inflicted by unavoidable medical procedures (e.g., intubation, suctioning) or secondary to gastroesophageal reflux, a multidisciplinary team consisting of a pediatrician or gastroenterologist, nutritionist, occupational therapist, and a psychiatrist or psychologist is best equipped to meet the needs of these infants.

Before the psychiatric intervention can begin, if the child has a medical condition that produced the trauma, such as gastroesophageal reflux, the illness needs to be addressed first, and the child needs to be relieved of pain while feeding. In addition, the child's nutritional status needs to be assessed, and a plan for adequate nutritional intake needs to be developed. The child's nutritional status will determine whether the child can be treated conservatively as an outpatient or whether the child requires tube feeding, hospitalization, or both.

Outpatient Treatment of Young Infants

The main goal of the psychiatric intervention is to help the infant or young child overcome the fear of feeding. In my clinical experience, young infants who suffer from gastroesophageal reflux and who have come to associate feeding with vomiting and pain, and consequently have become frightened to drink from the bottle, can often be treated as outpatients, if they drink from the bottle when asleep. I explain to the parents that the infant has become afraid of feeding from the bottle and consequently it is best for the infant not to see the bottle for a while. Then I advise the parents to develop a schedule of bottle feedings during the time when the infant is put down for the morning nap, the afternoon nap, the evening bedtime, and one feeding during the night. It is best to feed the infant in the transition to sleep, when the infant is drowsy, but still sucking vigorously (infants maintain a sucking reflex, when the nipple is put in their mouth, up to 10 months of age). Interestingly, in this twilight state, the infants seem to be very relaxed and can drink 4 to 6 ounces of milk without vomiting. However, if they wake up and see the bottle, they become frightened, and often stop drinking and bat the bottle away. On the other hand, if their reflux is successfully treated, and they have been feeding from the bottle in the twilight state for about a month, they may wake up, see the bottle, and continue feeding without being scared. Once they have reached this state, the bottle feedings can gradually be transitioned to waking times.

At the same time as the bottle feedings go on, the infants are introduced to spoon feedings. This should be done very slowly and carefully. The emphasis should be on making spoon feedings a pleasurable experience and not on how much calories the parent can get into the infant. In young infants, the bottle feedings should be the major source of caloric intake, and spoon feedings should be more of a practice experience. The danger is that infants become stressed and frightened of spoon feedings as well, and the whole feeding experience becomes a struggle between mother and child. Mothers need to be supported in understanding this concept because of their worry about the infant's caloric intake.

The following case illustrates the treatment of a young infant who refused to drink from the bottle when awake:

Example: Vivian was 15 weeks old when she was referred to the Multidisciplinary Feeding Disorders Team. The main concern was that she would cry upon seeing the bottle and arch her back when put in the feeding position. Her mother, Mrs. Brown, reported that the only way she could feed Vivian from the bottle was when she was asleep. This had started a few weeks previously, after Vivian had been spitting up quite a bit during and after feedings and vomited almost daily.

Vivian's birth history was unremarkable. She weighed 8 pounds and 3 ounces at birth, and was initially breast-fed. However, Vivian nursed for such long periods of time that Mrs. Brown preferred to pump her milk and bottle–feed Vivian. When Vivian was about 6 weeks old, she started to spit up during and after feedings and sometimes vomit. Mrs. Brown noticed that Vivian started to arch herself during feedings, and that she had to wrap Vivian tightly and feed her in a side position to facilitate better feedings. About 6 weeks previously, Mrs. Brown observed that Vivian was vomiting almost daily and gradually decreased her intake, and 3 weeks previously, she started to cry just at the sight of the bottle. She became so resistant to feedings that Mrs. Brown was unable to feed her any more when she was awake.

The nutritional assessment revealed that Vivian had grown well in spite of her feeding difficulties. She was at the 70th percentile for weight and length on the growth chart, and her head circumference was at the 85th percentile. However, her caloric intake was only 60% of the recommended daily allowance for her age.

The medical assessment confirmed the diagnosis of gastroesophageal reflux, and the oral motor assessment found that Vivian had a coordinated suck, swallow, and breathing pattern during feeding.

The observation of Vivian and her mother showed a happy baby until her mother positioned Vivian to start the feeding. Vivian cried the moment Mrs. Brown positioned her for feeding, and then arched herself and batted the bottle away. When Mrs. Brown put the bottle on the table and sat Vivian up in her lap, Vivian gradually calmed, but cried even louder when her mother made a second attempt to feed her. Mrs. Brown gave up and walked around the room with Vivian on her shoulder until Vivian finally settled. After a while Vivian fell asleep in her mother's arms and drank all 6 ounces of milk in the bottle.

The team explained to Mr. and Mrs. Brown that Vivian had gastroesophageal reflux and had developed a Posttraumatic Feeding Disorder, that she seemed to have made an association between feeding from the bottle and pain and vomiting, and that she had become afraid of feeding.

Vivian was given medication for her reflux, and it was recommended that Mrs. Brown feed Vivian only during her transitions to sleep, when she was put down for her morning nap, her afternoon nap, at bedtime, and one or two times during the night. Because Vivian had such a strong reaction to seeing the bottle, it was recommended that Mrs. Brown not let her see the bottle for a while.

In addition, Mrs. Brown was encouraged to start spoon feedings two or three times daily to expose Vivian to another mode of feeding. It was explained to the parents that Vivian was getting enough milk from her "sleep feedings" and that they should think of the spoon feedings as practice sessions that should be pleasurable and not meant to get calories into Vivian at this point in time.

At the 2-week follow-up session, the parents reported that the medication seemed to be effective, that Vivian took her sleep feedings very well without any spitting up or vomiting. A few times, she had awakened during the feedings and pushed the bottle away, but she did not cry. Vivian was slow to get used to the spoon feedings; she seemed not to know what to do with the food, and most of it seemed to fall out of her mouth. However, she seemed to like the experience and would accept the spoon without resistance. The parents were greatly relieved that feedings were not such a struggle anymore.

They came back for another follow-up, when Vivian was 6 months old. By this time, Vivian was still getting her bottle feedings when going to sleep, but if she woke up and saw the bottle, she touched it without distress and would continue feeding while awake. She had also made nice progress with her spoon feedings and would eat up to a full baby jar of pureed food three times a day. Her growth had progressed nicely along the 80th percentiles, and the parents felt relieved that Vivian was making such nice progress.

When Vivian was about 8 months old, the parents reported that she transitioned to drinking from the bottle when awake. She continued to make progress eating her baby food, and at 10 months of age was started on soft table food. She learned to walk independently at 11 months of age and outgrew her gastroesophageal reflux when she was 1 year old.

Outpatient Treatment of Toddlers and Young Children

Toddlers or young children who have had an episode of severe gagging or choking or have been force-fed and consequently develop a Posttraumatic Feeding Disorder usually present with refusal to eat any solid food but are willing to drink from the bottle or glass and may accept finely pureed food that they can easily swallow. These children have an intense fear of swallowing any food that requires chewing. They often refuse any solid food, and if they allow any food to enter their mouth, they may pocket it and spit it out later. For these children I have developed a gradual desensitization method that allows them to overcome their fear of swallowing.

At baseline, it is important that the nutritional requirements of these children are taken care of by their bottle feedings and that the parents are helped to develop a regular feeding schedule with meals (including the bottle feedings) to be scheduled 3 to 4 hours apart, to allow the child to become hungry. Meals start with feedings of purees, if the child accepts them, and the purees are very gradually thickened over time. The parent should use two spoons and encourage the child to self-feed because this will occupy the child and make him or her less vigilant about the food. At the beginning, it can also be helpful to play soft music or to allow the child to look at television as a distraction and make him or her less fearful (this is the only feeding disorder for which distractions should be used to help the children to be less vigilant about the food the parents put in their mouth). Children who do not accept any purees should be offered very soft finger foods that melt in their mouth. The parent should eat the same foods and model for the child how to chew and swallow the food. Toddlers are very observant of what their parents eat and are more likely to put a food in their mouth if the parent eats it. The parents should give the toddler only a few pieces at a time to keep him or her from pocketing the food. The parent should not give the toddler any food that is hard to chew, even if the toddler asks for it. The parents should say, "You need to learn to chew better before you can eat this food." Toddlers with a Posttraumatic Feeding Disorder are often delayed in their ability to maneuver food in their mouth because of their lack of experience, and they are at risk of swallowing the food without much chewing and then gag or choke on it.

The feedings should be very relaxed and joyful, and there should be no pressure regarding how much the toddler actually eats. At the end of the feeding, the toddler should be given the bottle with an age-appropriate milk formula that supplies the nutritional needs of the child. However, there should be no bottle feedings outside of these scheduled mealtimes. Through modeling by the parents, by allowing the toddler to self-feed, and by increasing the texture of the food very gradually, these toddlers become increasingly confident and overcome their fear of eating solid food.

The following case illustrates this treatment method:

Example: Adam presented to the Feeding Disorders Clinic when he was 2½ years old because about 6 weeks previously he had started to refuse any solid food and became distressed if his parents urged him to eat his regular diet, which included all kinds of solid food. Since then, he had been taking only drinkable yogurts, ice cream, and an enriched breakfast drink. Occasionally, he licked some peanut butter off the spoon. This behavior started when his parents, Mr. and Mrs. Johnson, had explained to him that he was going to preschool soon. He asked a lot of questions, seemed quite anxious anticipating the new experience, had difficulty going to bed, and would wake up at night and come into his parents' bed. Around this time, he also had some molars breaking through, and one evening, he gagged on some food that he had been eating before without difficulty. The parents did not think much of it, but the next day, Adam took only very little bites of his food, and the following day refused to eat anything that had to be chewed. He also went through a period of being fearful of his bath, which he had previously enjoyed. In spite of his anticipatory anxiety, he had gone to preschool, and after a few days, was able to separate from his parents without much difficulty. In the last 2 weeks, he seemed more relaxed and had started to lick peanut butter off the spoon.

His birth history and early feeding development were unremarkable. He had never been a big eater but grew along the 20th percentile for weight and height and the 50th percentile for head circumference. He had always been a very cautious and perceptive little boy with excellent cognitive and speech development.

The medical assessment did not reveal any medical issues that had to be addressed. The oral motor assessment showed effective tongue and lip movements and impressive speech and language skills. The nutritional assessment showed a good growth pattern and adequate caloric intake from the liquid foods that he was able to eat.

The psychiatric assessment, which included the observation of Adam and his parents from behind a one-way mirror during a lunch meal and during play, showed a very bright and talkative little boy until it came to lunch, when he had trouble staying in his chair and started to cry every time his parents encouraged him to try some of the foods that they were eating. However, he recovered when they gave him his yogurt and ice cream. During the play, he enjoyed feeding the boy doll all kinds of play food, and the psychiatrist talked with him about how "the little boy doll was not scared to eat."

The psychiatrist on the team explained to Mr. and Mrs. Johnson that Adam seemed to have been rather anxious in anticipation of going to preschool, when he gagged on solid food, and consequently he developed a severe fear of eating solid food that needed to be chewed and swallowed. As he seemed otherwise healthy and was getting adequate calories from the drinkable foods that he was taking, the emphasis of the treatment should be on helping him overcome his fear of eating solids by gradually introducing him to purees and foods of increasing consistency. The occupational therapist gave the parents a list of soft finger foods that would easily melt in his mouth. The parents were encouraged to give him only very small amounts of the purees and the soft finger food and wait for Adam to ask for more. It was suggested that they start with one kind of a pureed food that Adam used to like and for them to eat the same food in order for Adam to see that his parents were comfortable eating the food. Once he was comfortable to eat one type of a pureed food, they could start offering him another pureed food of a somewhat thicker consistency and gradually move to a greater variety of pureed foods. Once Adam was comfortable with thicker purees, they could start offering him just one or two pieces of the melt-away finger foods and let him pace himself as to how much he wanted to eat of the different foods. They could encourage him by saying that he did a good job chewing and swallowing his food, but they should not make too much of a deal by clapping when he ate, because this can make some children too self-conscious about their eating and make them more anxious.

When Adam and his parents came for their follow-up appointment 2 weeks later, Adam was feeding himself yogurt and had started to eat some applesauce. He still seemed anxious during the meal and would move a lot in his chair, but with reminders he was able to stay in his chair, and he expressed interest in what else his parents were eating. After the meal, the psychiatrist played with Adam and his parents in the room with the boy doll and play food. Adam took great pleasure in serving everybody pretend pizza and chicken, and the therapist talked for the boy doll and said, "I have been scared to eat because I gagged, but now I can eat again, and I am not scared anymore." Adam listened intently and then gave the doll some more pizza.

Adam was seen every 3 to 4 weeks. He continued to make gradual progress and started to eat food with increased texture, meats being the last on his list. After 3 months, Adam was back to eating his regular diet.

Various Treatments of Severe Feeding Resistance

As illustrated in the cases above, infants and toddlers who are in no nutritional danger because they are drinking from the bottle or accepting pureed food from the spoon can be treated as outpatients. However, some infants and young children are so resistant to eat or drink in any form that they require tube feedings in order to survive. Unfortunately, the tube feedings further blunt the children's appetite and often intensify the children's food refusal.

A few studies have been published on how to help these children to overcome their feeding resistance and to learn to eat again. Benoit, Wang, and Zlotkin (2000) conducted a study of 64 children ranging in age from 4 to 36 months who were tube fed and showed severe feeding resistance. All children were put on a regular meal schedule to stimulate the hunger/satiety cycle, and half of the children were randomized to receive in addition behavioral extinction therapy. Extinction is defined as removing the reinforcer to a response (e.g., removing the spoon after the child's refusal to open her mouth negatively reinforces the food refusal, whereas nonremoval of the spoon is an extinction procedure). Extinction consisted of gently placing a small amount of food directly on the lips or inside the mouth of the child. This usually triggered a distress response in the child. The feeder actively reassured the child when he or she became anxious or agitated as the food was offered and gently placed a new spoonful of food on the lips or inside the mouth every 5 to 10 seconds despite the child's distress. Feeding in this manner continued so that the child's experience was that gagging or food refusal did not stop the feeding. In addition, operant conditioning techniques, such as praise (e.g., "good bite," "good swallow"), were also used. However, the authors felt that operant conditioning techniques alone were unhelpful to treat traumatically acquired resistance to feeding.

During seven weekly sessions, the therapist modeled for the primary feeders of the child the behavioral technique described above, and the primary feeders were instructed to practice the behavioral techniques at home between sessions. Before treatment, and if the child gained weight or the weight remained stable during the previous week, the primary feeder was instructed to reduce the volume of tube feeding by 25%. If the child lost weight during the previous week, then the volume of the tube feeding was increased by 25%. At follow-up, half of the children in behavioral therapy and none of the children in the control group were no longer tube-dependent. However, this behavioral treatment program requires skillful handling of the child by the therapist and the parent because it can easily turn into force-feeding and further traumatize the child.

Behavioral techniques for inpatient treatment of these children have been described by Babbitt and colleagues (1994) and more recently by Linscheid (2006). Linscheid pointed out that treatment of feeding problems in children involves two major components—

appetite manipulation and contingency management—and that success of treatment relies on the child's motivation to change his or her current eating pattern. In toddlers and young children, motivation is directly related to deprivation of calories. Whereas specific behavioral procedures are important in treatment, Linscheid believed that inducing hunger in the child is almost always as important for success as (if not more than) the specific behavioral contingencies utilized. Typically, for an inpatient admission, for the first day or two, while supplying water or Pedialyte, any caloric formula feedings through the child's tube are stopped. As treatment progresses, it is determined on a day-to-day basis, depending on the child's weight loss, whether calories need to be delivered via the feeding tube to ensure that the child does not lose too much weight. If necessary, calories are given through tubes only at night in order to break the connection in the child's mind between feedings via the tube and hunger cessation.

The treatment is done by trained therapists three times a day, 7 days a week, and consists of behavioral contingencies in the feeding situation, a straightforward manipulation of reinforcing consequences to the child's behavior. The most commonly utilized positive reinforcers are social praise and social interaction, access to preferred toys or favorite videos, and access to preferred foods. Behaviors that interfere with feeding, such as pushing the spoon away, crying, or turning the head away, are treated by mild punishment in the form of a brief time-out. The feeder withdraws the food and physically turns away from the child, which constitutes a time-out from positive reinforcement. Some negative reinforcement procedures are also used. One such procedure involves the therapist holding a loaded spoon at the child's lip until the mouth is opened and the food accepted, or the child has to finish the food before getting out of the high chair. However, Linscheid (2006) warned that the therapist needs to be prepared to sit with the child until the food is finished, and that failing to realize the importance of follow-through with these contingencies can be a major cause of treatment failure.

Initially, the parent is absent from the treatment room. When treatment gains have been made and the therapist is confident that the techniques are working, the parent is brought into the room to observe the therapist during meals. This may result in loss of some previous gains the child made, but the progress is quickly made up when the child realizes that the contingencies have not changed even though the parent is in the room. The therapist explains to the parent the social praise and withdrawal of attention contingent on the child's behavior, and the next step is that the parent feeds the child with the therapist in a coaching role. The final step is to have the parent feed the child with the therapist nearby behind a one-way mirror. The children are generally discharged when three criteria are met: The first is that the child is taking sufficient calories to at least maintain his or her weight. The second is that the initial treatment goals are achieved, and the third discharge criterion is that the parents feel they are sufficiently familiar with the techniques and able to implement them at home. Cook, Linscheid, Rasnake, and Lukens (2000) report that by using this intervention they were able to achieve an 87.9% success rate for elimination of feeding tubes, with an average length of stay of only 8.77 days.

Duniz and colleagues (1996) have also described a successful inpatient treatment for infants and young children who are dependent on tube-feeding because of severe feeding resistance. The infants and their parents are admitted to a psychosomatic unit with a multidisciplinary team who oversees the infant's physical health and works with the parents and child in psychotherapy and play therapy. Tube feedings are discontinued, and parents and staff are given two basic rules: (a) offer the infant food if, and only if, a hunger cue has been shown, and (b) stop feeding immediately after any hint of refusal of food. The infants are offered food at intervals to experiment with, and as they experience hunger they begin to approach food and within days begin to eat independently. The authors report that the psychotherapeutic work with the parents fosters a healthier parent–child relationship and reduces parental psychopathology.

There have been a few case reports of the treatment of this disorder with low-dose selective serotonin reuptake inhibitors (SSRIs). Banerjee, Bhandari, and Rosenberg (2005) described 3 children, ranging in age from 7 to 12 years, diagnosed with choking phobia who were refractory to prior interventions and showed a rapid and sustained improvement with a low dose of an SSRI. In addition, Celik, Diler, Tahiroglu, and Avci (2007) described 24-month-old twins with a Posttraumatic Feeding Disorder who, when 3 months old, underwent several gastrointestinal procedures. After the hospitalization, they refused all solid food and some liquids and became tube-dependent. At age 2, they were started on fluoxetine 5 mg per day to treat their anxiety and fear about feeding. After 1 month, the children showed a significant decrease in anxiety during feeding and could be fed without requiring the feeding tube. The children showed no side effects to the medication.

In summary, each child with a Posttraumatic Feeding Disorder needs to be assessed to determine which treatment is most appropriate for the child and his or her family.

Differential Diagnosis and Comorbidities

This feeding disorder needs to be differentiated from Infantile Anorexia and from food refusal because of Sensory Food Aversions. Both disorders are described in detail in other chapters of this book. Infantile Anorexia is characterized by an inconsistent pattern of food refusal depending on the mood of the child. Anorectic children are not afraid to eat and can eat all types of food. Sensory Food Aversions usually involve foods with a certain taste, texture, temperature, and/or smell. Usually, the food refusal by the child is selective and not as global as seen in a Posttraumatic Feeding Disorder. Children with Sensory Food

Aversions will eat well if they are offered their preferred foods. However, sometimes children with Sensory Food Aversions develop a Posttraumatic Feeding Disorder if they experience a strong aversive reaction to a food, such as gagging or vomiting, and they generalize their fear to other foods that remind them of the aversive food. Children with Infantile Anorexia and those with Sensory Food Aversions can develop a Posttraumatic Feeding Disorder if the parents resort to force-feeding, especially if they force the child to eat aversive foods that trigger gagging and vomiting.

In addition, Posttraumatic Feeding Disorder needs to be differentiated from a Feeding Disorder Associated With a Concurrent Medical Condition (which is described in chapter 7). As illustrated in the cases above, infants with gastroesophageal reflux can develop a Posttraumatic Feeding Disorder that may mask the underlying medical condition. It is very important to get a good feeding and medical history to determine what triggered the fear of eating in the child. If the feeding difficulties were initially characterized by arching and crying during feeding and then progressed to distress in anticipation of feeding and food refusal, the child may have "silent" gastroesophageal reflux that was not recognized because the child did not vomit. Vomiting is usually the leading symptom of this medical condition, and children who have regurgitation secondary to gastroesophageal reflux but do not vomit are sometimes not diagnosed. In any case, the diagnosis of Posttraumatic Feeding Disorder is often associated with other feeding disorders and with medical conditions.

References

Babbitt, R. L., Hoch, T. A., Coe, D. A., Cataldo, M. F., Kelly, K. J., Stackhouse, C., & Perman, J. A. (1994). Behavioral assessment and treatment of pediatric feeding disorders. *Journal of Developmental and Behavioral Pediatrics, 15*, 278–291.

Banerjee, S. P., Bhandari, R. P., & Rosenberg, D. R. (2005). Use of low-dose selective serotonin reuptake inhibitors for severe, refractory choking phobia in childhood. *Journal of Developmental and Behavioral Pediatrics, 26*, 123–127.

Benoit, D., Wang, E. E., & Zlotkin, S. H. (2000). Discontinuation of enterostomy tube feeding by behavioral treatment in early childhood: A randomized controlled trial. *The Journal of Pediatrics, 137*, 498–503.

Celik, G., Diler, R. S., Tahiroglu, A. Y., & Avci, A. (2007). Fluoxetine in posttraumatic eating disorder in two-year-old twins. *Journal of Child and Adolescent Psychopharmacology, 17*, 233–236.

Chatoor, I. (1991). Eating and nutritional disorders of infancy and early childhood. In J. Wiener (Ed.), *Textbook of child and adolescent psychiatry* (pp. 351–361). Washington, DC: American Psychiatric Press.

Chatoor, I., & Ammaniti, M. (2007). A classification of feeding disorders of infancy and early childhood. In W. E. Narrow, M. B. First, P. Sirovatka, & D. A. Regier (Eds.), *Age and gender considerations in psychiatric diagnosis: A research agenda for DSM-V* (pp. 227–242). Arlington, VA: American Psychiatric Press.

Chatoor, I., Conley, C., & Dickson, L. (1988). Food refusal after an incident of choking: A posttraumatic eating disorder. *Journal of the American Academy of Child and Adolescent Psychiatry, 27*, 105–110.

Chatoor, I., Ganiban, J., Harrison, J., & Hirsch, R. (2001). Observation of feeding in the diagnosis of posttraumatic feeding disorder of infancy. *Journal of the American Academy of Child and Adolescent Psychiatry, 40*, 595–602.

Cook, C. M., Linscheid, T. R., Rasnake, I. K., & Lukens, C. T. (2000, April). *Long term followup of pediatric patients treated for feeding problems.* Paper presented at the North Coast Regional Conference, Society of Pediatric Psychology, Cleveland, OH.

de Lucas-Taracena, M. T., & Montañés-Rada, F. (2006). Swallowing phobia: Symptoms, diagnosis, and treatment. *Actas Españolas de Psiquiatría, 34*, 309–316.

Dellert, S. F., Hyams, J. S., Treem, W. R., & Geertsma, M. A. (1993). Feeding resistance and gastroesophaeal reflux in infancy. *Journal of Pediatric Gastroenterology and Nutrition, 17*(1), 66–71.

Duniz, M., Scheer, P. J., Trojovsky, A., Kaschnitz, W., Kvas, E., & Macari, S. (1996). Changes in psychopathology of parents of NOFT (non-organic failure to thrive) infants during treatment. *European Child & Adolescent Psychiatry, 5*, 93–100.

Kaplan, P. R., & Evans, I. M. (1978). A case of functional dysphagia treated on the model of fear. *Journal of Behavior Therapy and Experimental Psychiatry, 9*, 71–72.

Liebowitz, M. R. (1987). Globus hystericus and panic attacks. *The American Journal of Psychiatry, 144*, 390–391.

Linscheid, T. R. (2006). Behavioral treatments for pediatric feeding disorders. *Behavior Modification, 30*(1), 6–23.

McNally, R. J. (1994). Choking phobia: Review of the literature. *Comprehensive Psychiatry, 35*, 83–89.

Narrow, W. E., First, M. B., Sirovatka, P., & Regier, D. A. (Eds.). (2007). *Age and gender considerations in psychiatric diagnosis: A research agenda for DSM-V.* Arlington, VA: American Psychiatric Press.

Scheeringa, M., Anders, T., Boris, N., Carter, A., Chatoor, I., Egger, H., et al. (2003). Research diagnostic criteria for infants and preschool children: The process and empirical support. *Journal of the American Academy of Child and Adolescent Psychiatry 42*, 1504–1512.

Solyom, L., & Sookman, D. (1980). Fear of choking and its treatment: A behavioural approach. *Canadian Journal of Psychiatry, 25*, 30–34.

ZERO TO THREE. (2005). *Diagnostic classification of mental health and developmental disorders of infancy and early childhood: Revised edition (DC:0–3R).* Washington, DC: Author.

7

FEEDING DISORDER ASSOCIATED WITH A CONCURRENT MEDICAL CONDITION

Nosology

Failure to thrive (FTT), which has been equated with feeding disorders in infants and young children, was initially believed to be caused either by organic problems or nonorganic causes (e.g., maternal deprivation). In 1981, Homer and Ludwig described a third category of FTT, a mixed type that is caused by a combination of various organic and nonorganic problems. Since then, it has been accepted that organic conditions can be complicated by psychological difficulties and lead to severe feeding problems and growth failure. However, the specific feeding difficulties seen in infants and young children with medical conditions have not been well defined. The diagnostic criteria that I describe below address common feeding problems associated with gastroesophageal reflux and respiratory or cardiac conditions that compromise the infant's or young child's food intake. The diagnostic criteria listed below were included in *Diagnostic Classification of Mental Health and Developmental Disorders of Infancy and Early Childhood: Revised Edition (DC:0–3R;* ZERO TO THREE, 2005) and were described in Chatoor and Ammaniti's (2007) chapter in *Age and Gender Considerations in Psychiatric Diagnosis: A Research Agenda for DSM-V* (Narrow, First, Sirovatka, & Regier, 2007).

Diagnostic Criteria

A. This feeding disorder is characterized by food refusal and inadequate food intake for at least 2 weeks.

B. The onset of the food refusal can occur at any age of the child and may wax and wane in intensity, depending on the underlying medical condition.

C. The infant or toddler readily initiates feeding, but over the course of feeding, shows distress and refuses to continue feeding.

D. The infant or toddler has a concurrent medical condition that is believed to cause the distress (e.g., gastroesophageal reflux, or cardiac or respiratory disease).

E. The infant or toddler fails to gain adequate weight or may even lose weight.

F. Medical management improves but may not fully alleviate the feeding problems.

Clinical Presentation

Infants with respiratory distress or cardiac disease may feed for a while and take a few ounces until they tire out and stop feeding. In general, the feeding difficulties of these infants lead to inadequate food intake, failure to gain weight, or loss of weight. These feeding difficulties are more easily recognized, whereas some medical conditions are not readily diagnosed, and for those, food refusal may be the leading symptom. For example, food allergies can be difficult to diagnose in infants, and "silent" gastroesophageal reflux without vomiting can be overlooked because regurgitation and vomiting are usually the leading symptoms that alert pediatricians to this condition. I have observed that infants with reflux may drink 1 to 2 ounces of milk before the reflux seems to become activated. The infants then signal distress by arching and crying, and refuse to continue feeding. Some infants can be calmed and resume feeding, but others may become increasingly agitated while their caretakers continue to offer the bottle or food.

Several authors have described that feeding problems and maternal distress are commonly seen in infants with gastroesophageal reflux. Shepherd, Wren, Evans, Lander, and Ong (1987) reported that feeding difficulties and dysphagia were seen in 44% of the infants with gastroesophageal reflux they studied. In addition, excessive crying, irritability, and sleep disturbances were the most common symptoms. Although it has been well recognized that silent gastroesophageal reflux can be associated with serious respiratory symptoms, such as microaspiration of the refluxate or reflex bronchospasm, and a number of other airway symptoms, such as recurrent croup, wheezing, blue spells, and hoarseness, Carr and colleagues (2000) pointed out that feeding symptoms, including choking/gagging, food refusal, and arching, as well as FTT, are important symptoms of gastroesophageal reflux. Heine, Jordan, Lubitz, Meehan, and Catto-Smith (2006) reported that 56% of parents whose infants had gastroesophageal reflux described their infant to be difficult to feed. Many refused feedings when hungry, and back arching was reported by the parents in 57%

of the infants. Feeding difficulties and back arching were significantly more common in infants younger than 3 months.

Whereas back arching is frequently described in the very young infants, Mathisen, Worrall, Masel, Wall, and Shepherd (1999) drew attention to oral motor dysfunction in 16 of 20 infants with gastroesophageal reflux with a mean age of 6 months. Compared to a control group, these infants showed significantly more food refusal, had fewer self-feeding skills and readiness behaviors for solids, more immature tongue and jaw control, and more food loss. There were more panic reactions and choking episodes observed in these infants and developmental delays in self-feeding, such as holding the spoon. These infants were significantly more demanding, had fewer vocalizations, and were more difficult to feed.

In summary, these studies indicate that feeding difficulties are frequently associated with gastroesophageal reflux. Arching, crying, and food refusal in very young infants, and gagging and immature oral motor skills combined with resistance to feeding in older infants, should alert the clinician to consider reflux in the differential diagnosis of feeding difficulties, especially if the presenting symptom is food refusal. A diagnostic study (Chatoor et al., 2003) showed that this feeding disorder can be diagnosed with high interrater reliability, when both diagnosticians based their diagnosis on the feeding history, as given by the mother, and the observation of mother–infant interactions during feeding. However, without the observation of the feeding, a third diagnostician missed the diagnosis in one third of the cases.

The following case illustrates the feeding difficulties described above in a young infant with gastroesophageal reflux:

Example: Joan was 8 months old when she was referred to the Multidisciplinary Feeding Disorders Team because of eating only small amounts of food and poor weight gain. Her mother, Mrs. Smith, reported that Joan would drink only small amounts of milk and eat very little most days. Sometimes, she would drink a whole bottle of milk at night, but usually during the day she would not accept more than 2 ounces at a time before she would cry and refuse to take any more. When offered pureed baby foods, she would move it around her mouth and lose most of it. She was a happy baby in general, but she cried a lot during feedings. Mrs. Smith felt exhausted because feeding would take more than an hour, and she felt that she was feeding Joan all day long without getting much food into her.

Joan was the product of a full-term normal pregnancy and delivery and weighed 6 pounds and 5 ounces at birth. Mrs. Smith felt that Joan fed well for the first 2 months, although she never took more than 4 to 5 ounces of formula at a time. She had some wet burps, but only occasionally vomited. These feeding behaviors changed when Joan was about 2 months old. She started to cry during feedings and would often arch herself so that her mother had to stop the feeding. Because she gained weight so slowly, her pediatrician changed her to an enriched formula to boost her calories. However, Joan continued to take only small amounts of the new formula, and her crying during feedings became more intense. She also started to vomit more often. At 6 months of age, her pediatrician prescribed an antacid, but Mrs. Smith stopped it after 3 weeks because Joan's feeding behavior and food intake did not improve, and Joan resisted taking the medicine.

The nutritional assessment revealed that Joan's weight was below the 5th percentile and her height at the 10th percentile, giving her 85% of her ideal body weight and placing her in the range of mild malnutrition. The oral motor assessment showed that Joan was somewhat delayed in her ability to handle solid food, and at the age of 8 months had the oral motor skills of a 6–month-old infant. Her overall muscle tone was also low, and she had difficulty sitting independently for any length of time, which made feeding in the high chair stressful for her.

The observation of mother and infant during feeding and play from behind a one-way mirror showed mutually pleasurable interactions between Mrs. Smith and Joan before the feeding. However, when placed in the high chair, Joan looked distressed. She had difficulty keeping herself upright and was sliding down in the high chair while her mother tried to feed her some pureed food. When Joan started crying, Mrs. Smith took her out of the high chair and placed her in her lap to give her the bottle. Joan took the bottle willingly, but after a few minutes started to arch herself and pushed the bottle away. Mrs. Smith waited for a few minutes and let Joan touch the bottle and play with it before she offered it again. Joan accepted the bottle again, but a few minutes later, stopped suckling, pushed the bottle away, and started to cry more intensely. She did not recover from her crying for more than 10 minutes, and Mrs. Smith gave up trying to feed her anymore.

These behaviors seemed characteristic of a baby who was experiencing pain during feedings, and consequently, the gastroenterologist on the team initiated a medical work-up for gastroesophageal reflux, which confirmed the diagnosis.

Course of Feeding Disorder

As indicated in the case described above, untreated gastroesophageal reflux can cause much distress to the infant and also to the parents who try to feed their crying and arching babies. An early study by Shepherd and colleagues (1987) reported that in spite of the severe symptoms during early infancy, 55% of the infants they studied were symptom-free at 10 months of age, and 81% were symptom-free by 18 months of age. However, some infants continued to have symptoms of reflux, and some children had severe disease that required surgery. A 1-year follow-up study of gastroesophageal reflux by Nelson, Chen, Syniar, and Christoffel (1998), who first diagnosed the infants when they were 6 to 12 months of age, reported that at follow-up the parents were more likely than those of control subjects to report frequent food refusal, that it usually took more than an hour for the child to eat his or her meals, and that it was upsetting to the parents to think about meals. In his review, Gold (2004) noted that in the absence of longitudinal studies with well-defined cases and controls, and studies of adults who recalled symptoms of reflux as children, it is likely that children with gastroesophageal reflux may become adults with reflux.

Considering the findings from these studies and understanding that specific feeding problems, such as crying during feedings, arching, and refusing to continue feeding after having taken only a small amount of milk or food, can be early signs of gastroesophageal reflux, the clinician should intervene early and treat the underlying medical condition to prevent long-term symptoms. In my own clinical work, I have seen young infants with reflux associating feeding with pain and becoming so afraid of feeding that they cried at the sight of the bottle and refused to have the nipple of the bottle put in his or her mouth. I have described this outcome in more detail in the previous chapter on Posttraumatic Feeding Disorder.

Etiology

Although young infants cannot verbalize their feelings, they express themselves through crying and through their body language. In observing infants and their mothers during feeding, I have come to respect how sensitive some infants are, and how strongly they express their distress through crying and arching away from their caretakers. Gastroesophageal reflux is known to cause heartburn in adults and seems to cause pain and severe distress in infants as well. In my observation, infants express their pain and distress by arching, crying, and refusing to feed.

Some studies have addressed the etiology of gastroesophageal reflux. A twin study from Sweden by Cameron and colleagues (2002) found increased concordance for reflux in monozygotic twins as compared to dizygotic twins, indicating a genetic rather than an environmental etiology. Orenstein and colleagues (2002) localized an autosomal dominant infantile gastroesophageal reflux gene on Chromosome 9. Although these studies indicate that reflux is a heritable condition, early intervention can have a strong impact on the severity of symptoms and the distress caused to the child and her family.

Treatment

Because of the interaction of organic and psychological factors contributing to the severe feeding difficulties of these children, collaboration between the pediatrician or pediatric specialist and the psychiatrist or psychologist is critical. Optimal medical treatment of the child's underlying illness is necessary before psychological interventions can be successful. Direct observation of infants with their primary caregivers during feeding is most helpful to understand the infants' and the parents' distress, and to monitor how well the medical condition is responding to the treatment. In addition, by videotaping the feedings and reviewing the tape with the parents, the therapist can problem solve with the parents and help them develop more appropriate strategies that allow infants to calm instead of escalating their distress during feeding.

However, in situations in which the medical illness cannot be adequately treated and the infant continues to experience distress during feedings and is unable to take in appropriate amounts of food for growth, supplemental nutrition through nasogastric or gastrostomy tubes must be considered. Then the therapist must work with the parents to maintain the infant's oral feeding skills while most of the nutrition is given via tube feedings. This can best be done by continuous feedings through the tube that is interrupted for 3 to 4 hours before oral feedings. According to the nutritional state of the infant, these oral feedings should be at a minimum of once daily or ideally two or three times daily, if the remaining tube feedings are adequate to provide the infant with the nutrients needed. During the oral feedings, the emphasis should be on making feeding a pleasant, enjoyable experience for the infant without paying attention to how much the infant actually eats.

As pointed out earlier and described in the case study above, some infants become malnourished and weak, with poor muscle tone and delayed oral motor development, which interferes with their ability to take in age-appropriate foods. In these situations, an occupational therapist can help the parents find appropriate seating for the child and choose foods that the child can actually handle without the danger of gagging and choking.

Through this multidisciplinary team work, the parents can learn to make feeding a pleasurable experience for the infant and guide the infant to acquire age-appropriate feeding skills. Again, reviewing the videotape of the infant's feeding and discussing the infant's cues with the parents is usually beneficial in sorting out how to best help the infant. In general, these are very difficult cases that require individualized attention by an experienced multidisciplinary team.

The following example describes a young infant who had "silent reflux" but was diagnosed early and responded well to the combination of medical and psychiatric intervention:

Example: Paul was 6 months old when he was referred by his pediatrician to the Multidisciplinary Feeding Disorders Clinic because of severe food refusal and poor growth. Mrs. Jones, his mother, reported that since birth Paul had occasionally spit up a little during and after feedings, but during the previous 6 weeks, he had become increasingly difficult to feed. Mrs. Jones reported that Paul usually took 1 or 2 ounces of his formula and then would push the nipple out from his mouth and start to cry. If she tried to continue feeding Paul, he cried more intensely and became increasingly agitated until she comforted him by holding him on her shoulder and walking with him. Sometimes after walking him for 10 to 20 minutes, Mrs. Jones could resume feeding him, but often he started to cry again after only briefly sucking from the bottle. Mrs. Jones described that at night, Paul would wake up and cry as if he were hungry, but then he would take only a few ounces of milk and cry again. Mrs. Jones felt exhausted because she was trying to feed Paul day and night, but despite her efforts, Paul would drink only half of the formula that he was supposed to and had started to lose weight.

The nutritional evaluation revealed that Paul was only 84% of his ideal body weight, which put him in the range of mild malnutrition. His oral motor evaluation showed that his oral motor skills were slightly delayed, but Paul had good sucking movements and was able to handle baby purees without difficulty. The observation of feeding revealed pleasant mother–infant interactions at the beginning of the feeding, but after a few minutes of suckling, Paul pushed the nipple of the bottle out of his mouth, arched his back, and started to cry when his mother tried to get him back to feeding. The harder she tried, the more agitated Paul became, and mother and baby looked very distressed and gave up feeding. These feeding interactions raised concerns that Paul experienced gastroesophageal reflux that caused him pain and interfered with his feeding.

Further medical testing confirmed the diagnosis of moderate gastroesophageal reflux, which was somewhat surprising to the pediatrician and the gastroenterologist because Paul had not shown any vomiting, the most common symptom of reflux.

Paul was treated with medications for reflux, and his food intake doubled quickly. However, Mrs. Jones reported that if he drank more than 3 or 4 ounces at a time, the symptoms recurred. Mr. Jones videotaped mother and baby during feeding, and the therapist reviewed the videotape with both parents. The videotape showed clearly what Mrs. Jones had reported, that after having taken about 4 ounces of milk, Paul began to push the bottle away and started to arch himself. This information was shared with the gastroenterologist, who increased the dose of the reflux medication. Paul became more comfortable during feedings and tolerated up to 5 ounces of formula without showing any signs of distress. Once Mrs. Jones understood the reason for Paul's food refusal, she also learned to ease Paul's feeding difficulties by thickening his formula, keeping him upright after feedings, and feeding him at more frequent intervals of about 3 hours. Gradually, Paul tolerated larger amounts of formula at each feeding and woke up less frequently at night. At 15 months old, Paul was found to have outgrown the gastroesophageal reflux, and he was able to feed himself an age-appropriate diet.

Differential Diagnosis

This feeding disorder needs to be differentiated from other feeding disorders characterized by food refusal—for example, Infantile Anorexia, Sensory Food Aversions, and Posttraumatic Feeding Disorder—which are described in more detail in other chapters of this book. Key to understanding this feeding disorder and differentiating it from other feeding disorders is the observation of feeding, which reveals that the infant usually initiates feeding without difficulty, and that mother and child engage in pleasant reciprocal interactions until the infant experiences distress and stops feeding. However, the infants with gastroesophageal reflux who make an association between feeding and pain may cry in anticipation of feedings, refuse all feedings, and develop a Posttraumatic Feeding Disorder.

References

Cameron, A. J., Lagergren, J., Henriksson, C., Nyren, O., Locke, G. R., 3rd, & Pedersen, N. L. (2002). Gastroesophageal reflux disease in monozygotic and dizygotic twins. *Gastroenterology, 122*, 55–59.

Carr, M. M., Nguyen, A., Nagy, M., Poje, C., Pizzuto, M., & Brodsky, L. (2000). Clinical presentation as a guide to the identification of GERD in children. *International Journal of Pediatric Otorhinolaryngology, 54*, 27–32.

Chatoor, I., Paez, L., Harrison, J., Surles, J., Beker, L., Simenson, R., & Hirsch, R. (2003, October). The reliability of diagnostic criteria for feeding disorders. Abstract in *Scientific Proceedings of the 50th Anniversary Meeting of the American Academy of Child and Adolescent Psychiatry* (pp. 156). Miami Beach, FL.

Chatoor, I., & Ammaniti, M. (2007). A classification of feeding disorders of infancy and early childhood. In W. E. Narrow, M. B. First, P. Sirovatka, & D. A. Regier (Eds.), *Age and gender considerations in psychiatric diagnosis: A research agenda for DSM-V* (pp. 227–242). Arlington, VA: American Psychiatric Press.

Gold, B. D. (2004). Review article: Epidemiology and management of gastro-oesophageal reflux in children. *Alimentary Pharmacology & Therapeutics, 19*(Suppl. 1), 22–27.

Heine, R. G., Jordan, B., Lubitz, L., Meehan, M., & Catto-Smith, A. G. (2006). Clinical predictors of pathological gastro-oesophageal reflux in infants with persistent distress. *Journal of Paediatrics and Child Health, 42*, 134–139.

Homer, C., & Ludwig, S. (1981). Categorization of etiology of failure to thrive. *American Journal of Diseases of Children, 135*, 848–851.

Mathisen, B., Worrall, L., Masel, J., Wall, C., & Shepherd, R.W. (1999). Feeding problems in infants with gastro-oesophageal reflux disease: A controlled study. *Journal of Paediatrics and Child Health, 35*, 163–169.

Narrow, W. E., First, M. B., Sirovatka, P., & Regier, D. A. (Eds.). (2007). *Age and gender considerations in psychiatric diagnosis: A research agenda for DSM-V.* Arlington, VA: American Psychiatric Press.

Nelson, S. P., Chen, E. H., Syniar, G. M., & Christoffel, K. K. (1998). One-year follow-up of symptoms of gastroesophageal reflux during infancy. *Pediatrics, 102*(6), e67.

Orenstein, S. R., Shalaby, T. M., Finch, R., Pfuetzer, R. H., De Vandry, S., Chensny, L. J., et al. (2002). Autosomal dominant infantile gastroesophageal reflux disease: Exclusion of a 13q14 locus in five well characterized families. *American Journal of Gastroenterology, 97*, 2725–2732.

Shepherd, R. W., Wren, J., Evans, S., Lander, M., & Ong, T. H. (1987). Gastroesophageal reflux in children: Clinical profile, course and outcome with active therapy in 126 cases. *Clinical Pediatrics, 26*(2), 55–60.

ZERO TO THREE. (2005). *Diagnostic classification of mental health and developmental disorders of infancy and early childhood: Revised edition (DC:0–3R).* Washington, DC: Author.

COMORBIDITIES AND COMPLEX FEEDING DISORDERS

Differential Diagnosis and Comorbidity of Infantile Anorexia and Sensory Food Aversions

CHILDREN WITH INFANTILE ANOREXIA and Sensory Food Aversions are often referred to as "picky eaters," and many authors do not make any distinction between the symptoms of the two disorders. However, as I have discussed in previous chapters, Infantile Anorexia and Sensory Food Aversions are two distinct feeding disorders with different symptomatology and a different course, and most important, they respond to different interventions. Infantile Anorexia is characterized by inconsistent food refusal; the child has a poor appetite and would rather play, walk around, or talk than eat; the child is not interested in eating and may eat a food one day but refuse it the next day; the poor food intake leads to poor growth. On the other hand, Sensory Food Aversions are characterized by selective food refusal; the child consistently refuses certain foods because of the taste, texture, or smell but will eat preferred foods; the refusal of whole food groups leads to dietary deficiencies (i.e., in vitamins, minerals, or protein), but the child's weight is not affected.

In a diagnostic study by Chatoor and colleagues (2007), out of 431 toddlers and young children, 159 met criteria for Sensory Food Aversions, 83 met criteria for Infantile Anorexia, and 63 were comorbid for Infantile Anorexia and Sensory Food Aversions. The remaining children carried different diagnoses. The diagnosis of the feeding disorders was made independently by three professionals, two psychiatrists and one nurse practitioner, who had good inter-rater agreement. This study demonstrated that the symptoms of the two feeding disorders can be differentiated and that both feeding disorders present most commonly in the pure form, but both feeding disorders can also be found together in the same child.

Why is this important? I am often told that if Infantile Anorexia and Sensory Food Aversions can occur in the same child, maybe they are just different expressions of the same disorder. As I have described in detail in the previous chapters on these two disorders, they have different manifestations and different courses, and based on some preliminary evidence, I believe that they have different etiologies. However, most importantly, they respond differently to different interventions. Infantile Anorexia, which is characterized by the lack of appetite and poor weight gain, responds to facilitating internal regulation of eating by allowing the child to get hungry, which I have described in detail under the treatment of Infantile Anorexia. However, children who have Sensory Food Aversions and refuse to eat certain foods because they are afraid that the foods will be aversive to them will not eat these foods if they are made hungry. Quite to the contrary, they will get very upset and starve rather than eat any food that they expect to be aversive. Several parents have reported to me that on the advice of professionals, they offered the children only foods that the rest of the family were eating. The children would go for days starving and would not touch any of the food offered to them. If a child has both feeding disorders, he will have a low hunger drive because of the Infantile Anorexia, and he will be even more prone to starve if hunger is supposed to cure the problem of food refusal because of Sensory Food Aversions.

In the following case, I will outline the symptoms of these two feeding disorders and how to treat both disorders simultaneously. I will write in parentheses which symptoms are characteristic for one or the other feeding disorder. I will comment on how to differentiate the two feeding disorders and explain which intervention is directed toward which of the two feeding disorders.

Example 1

Chief Complaints

Lucas was a 3½-year-old boy with a long history of feeding problems. His parents, Mr. and Mrs. Johnson, were very concerned about Lucas eating only small amounts of food and having a very limited diet. The foods he consumed included hot dogs, cheese, pudding, yogurt, french fries, dry cereal, popcorn, pretzels, and chips. If they offered him a new food, he would cry, become angry, and act as if the new food was going to hurt him. At times when they tried to force him to eat a new food, he would gag or pocket it in his mouth and spit it out later. *(The gagging, the food selectivity, and the fear of trying any new foods are classical symptoms of Sensory Food Aversions.)*

The parents were also concerned that Lucas never asked for food, and when offered food would eat only small amounts. *(These are classic symptoms of Infantile Anorexia.)*

The parents also described that it was difficult to get Lucas to sit at the table at mealtimes. First, he did not want to stop his play and come to sit down at the table. Then he would be in and out of his seat and run around the room instead of eating. *(Not wanting to come to the table and wanting to play instead of eating are characteristic of children with Infantile Anorexia, but getting up and running around the room instead of eating can be seen in children with both feeding disorders. Children with Infantile Anorexia seem to get satiated quickly and tend to get up and want to play instead of eating. Children with Sensory Food Aversions become anxious at the table. They are afraid of being offered food they do not want to eat, and they may not even want to look at the food or smell the food other family members are eating.)*

Past Medical, Feeding, and Developmental History

Lucas was born full-term, weighing 6 pounds and 13 ounces, and was delivered without any complications. He took his formula well, and at 4 months of age, baby cereal was introduced. However, Lucas refused to eat the cereal. He would grimace and then refuse to open his mouth. At 6 months of age, he was introduced to baby food, but again he would grimace and spit out most of the baby food except for the more sweet varieties. He gagged occasionally, especially when introduced to stage 3 baby foods, a mixture of puree with lumps of other food in it, and he refused to eat any more baby food after the gagging. At 9 months, Lucas was given table food, and baby foods were withdrawn in the hope that he would accept table foods. However, he did not accept the table foods and refused to go back to the few baby foods he had accepted before. Between 9 and 12 months of age, Lucas was taking only formula and refused all solid food. At 12 months, he was given an enriched formula, and new efforts were made by his mother, Mrs. Johnson, to get him interested in table food. Lucas started to put some table foods in his mouth but would spit them out without swallowing. At 15 months of age, Lucas began to accept crunchy snack foods but nothing else. For the next year until Lucas was more than 2 years old, he accepted only crunchy and salty snack foods, pretzels being his favorite. Gradually, Mrs. Johnson talked him into trying hot dogs, cheese, and french fries, and in the past few months, Lucas had started to eat dry cereal and pudding. *(This part of Lucas's feeding history—the grimacing, spitting out the food, the gagging on stage 3 baby food, and the subsequent food refusal—is rather typical of a child with Sensory Food Aversions.)*

In addition, Mr. and Mrs. Johnson were concerned that Lucas had never shown much interest in feeding. As soon as he became more mobile and was cruising around the room, it was hard to get him in the high chair and get any food into him. Initially, Mrs. Johnson had used distractions to keep him busy, but when he was around 9 months old and learned to walk, it became impossible to get him in the high chair, and for the next few months, Lucas lived on milk only. When Lucas was 12 months old, the parents got him back in the high chair with a lot of toys and television as distractions while trying to feed him some table food. Lucas refused to open his mouth for most of the foods or spit them out as mentioned earlier, but with a lot of trial and error, Mrs. Johnson got him interested in crunchy snack foods that he could feed himself. But even when given his favorite foods, after a few minutes in the high chair, in spite of the television and the toys to distract him, Lucas would start throwing the food and try to climb out of the chair. When Lucas got to be around 18 months old, Mrs. Johnson started to leave food out for him to take whenever he felt like eating, but that did not seem to work either. However, Mrs. Johnson had started to let Lucas drink milk from the bottle whenever he wanted when he was about 9 months old and refused all solid food, and she had allowed this to continue until the time of the evaluation. Although he had weaned himself from drinking from the bottle during the day when he was busy playing, Lucas was still drinking from the bottle at bedtime and when he went down for his nap in the afternoon. *(This part of the history—Lucas's lack of interest in feeding, his reluctance to go into the high chair, his throwing of even his favorite foods, his efforts to get out of the high chair after a few minutes, and his mother's use of distractions, leaving out the food, and letting the child eat or drink whenever he wanted—is typical for Infantile Anorexia.)*

In addition to his feeding difficulties, Lucas had shown some other areas of sensory problems. He never liked to touch food and get his hands messy. If any soft food got on his hands, he would stretch out his hands and cry until his mother wiped his hands. He did not want to walk on sand or grass, and he did not like his hair to be cut or have any labels on his clothing. In addition, he was bothered by loud noises, such as when the vacuum cleaner was turned on, a fire engine could be heard, or a plane was going overhead. He also had difficulty with smells and often did not want to sit at the table if his parents ate fish or broccoli. He had been assessed by an early intervention program and found to be delayed in his fine motor and speech development. Although his receptive speech was good, he had problems with articulation of certain letters. Because of these delays, Lucas had seen an occupational therapist and a hearing and speech specialist who had helped greatly with his difficulties, and he was discharged from treatment after a short time because he made significant progress and was able to meet appropriate developmental milestones for his age. *Problems in other sensory areas are often associated with Sensory Food Aversions. These problems can involve hypersensitivities to touch, to sound, to smell, or to lights. Toddlers who are hypersensitive to touch often avoid any wet foods that they experience as "messy" and consequently do not want to eat these foods or prefer that their parents feed them. I have seen 3- and 4-year-old children with Sensory Food Aversions who were still being fed by their parents. Another complication of Sensory Food Aversions comes from the children's avoidance of chewy foods, such as raw vegetables and meats. Children like Lucas often show a delay in oral motor development and have difficulty with articulation. However, early intervention, like in the case of Lucas, can help them with these developmental delays.*

Nutritional Assessment

Lucas had started out at the 75th percentile for weight and height in the first 6 months of life, but dropped to the 50th percentile for weight and the 60th percentile for height by 12 months of age, after he had gone through 3 months of living on the bottle only. He continued to spiral down on the growth chart and, at the time of the assessment, placed on the 25th percentile for height and at the 5th percentile for weight. He had tall parents, his father being more than 6 feet tall and his mother measuring 5 feet 7 inches. He had maintained fair linear growth, but he was a very thin little boy. Lucas's weight for height was below the 5th percentile, making him 82% of ideal body weight and putting him in the range of mild malnutrition. A 3-day food record revealed that Lucas was taking in only 40% of the recommended daily allowance for a child of his age and was not getting adequate amounts of calories and micronutrients for optimal growth. *The nutritional assessment showed the effects of Infantile Anorexia that had slowed his weight gain and put him in the range of mild malnutrition, and it revealed that his limited diet was not providing him with the necessary micronutrients for optimal growth, which is one of the impairment criteria for Sensory Food Aversions.*

Observation of Feeding and Play Behavior

Lucas was observed during a meal and play with his parents from behind a one-way mirror. During the meal, he accepted his regular foods, a hot dog and french fries, although he ate only a few bites, and then got up to look at what was behind the curtain in the room. His parents asked him to return to his seat, but when they asked him to have some of their chicken and vegetables, he got very upset, started to cry, and jumped out of his seat to hide in the corner of the room. Mrs. Johnson coaxed him back to have his pudding, but as soon as he finished the small cup of pudding, he was up again talking about the pictures and the clock on the wall. After about 10 minutes, the meal was over for Lucas. While his parents continued to eat their meal, he was buzzing around the room and entertaining himself by looking in the mirror and making faces.

Lucas looked very different during his play. He was calm and thoughtful in building with the blocks and directing the cars through a tunnel he had built. He was engaged with both of his parents and enjoyed give-and-take while playing with them. *The observation of the feeding and play highlighted symptoms of Infantile Anorexia, namely, Lucas's stopping to eat after only a few bites and being more interested in what was behind the curtain and the things on the wall than in eating his food. The feeding observation also revealed his fear of trying new foods and his anxiety during the meal, which are often seen in children with Sensory Food Aversions.*

Summary of Diagnostic Findings

The history of Lucas's feeding development, the observation of the feeding and play, and the nutritional assessment revealed symptoms that met criteria for both Infantile Anorexia and Sensory Food Aversions. The lack of hunger signals, eating very little, getting out of the chair and playing rather than eating, and the mild malnutrition are symptoms of Infantile Anorexia, whereas the difficulties with the introduction of various baby foods and table foods, the grimacing, spitting out the food, the gagging, and subsequent refusal to eat baby foods and table foods, the ongoing refusal and fear of trying any new foods, the restriction of Lucas's diet to a limited number of foods, and the inadequacy of his diet in essential micronutrients are all symptoms of Sensory Food Aversions.

Treatment of Both Feeding Disorders

Treatment of both feeding disorders was conducted in the following way:

Initial Recommendations

The first step of the intervention was to help the parents understand the complexity of Lucas's feeding problems. With the help of the parent handouts that are attached to this chapter, I explained to Mr. and Mrs. Johnson Lucas's symptoms of Infantile Anorexia and Sensory Food Aversions. I briefly shared with them that from the limited evidence we have at this point, I believe that each feeding disorder has a different etiology and that, in my experience, Infantile Anorexia and Sensory Food Aversions respond to different interventions.

Because Lucas had shown such severe fear of trying any of the parents' food and was so highly anxious during the meal, I recommended that as a first step in the treatment of his Sensory Food Aversions the parents offer Lucas only foods that he was comfortable with, and that they stop asking him whether he wanted to try any of their foods. In case he wanted to try any of their foods, they were to tell him that he could have a little piece of their food but that this was really Mommy's or Daddy's food. If he wanted more, they could give him another little piece without making a big deal out of it. I have found that when toddlers or young children are given only a little piece of a new food, and the parents stay neutral rather than pushing the food onto the child, the children are more willing to try new foods. When the children are in control, they are less anxious and fearful that the food will taste or feel bad.

My treatment goals for Lucas were to help him overcome his fear of new foods and for him to initiate trying some foods that his parents were eating. I told him that I understood that he was scared to try new foods because some foods had made him feel bad or made him gag, and that his parents would not make him eat any more of their food. However, if he saw them eating something he thought he might like, he could ask them and they would give him a little piece to try.

Then I asked the parents to come back for a 2-hour session without Lucas so we could go over the feeding guidelines that are designed to help Lucas learn to recognize hunger and fullness and to regulate his eating accordingly. *(This part of the treatment I have described in detail in the chapter on Infantile Anorexia.)*

In addition, the nutritionist recommended that instead of regular milk, the parents switch to an enriched formula that would provide Lucas with the micronutrients which he did not get from his limited diet. The nutritionist also recommended that they stop giving him juice, because it was filling him up without providing him with adequate calories or micronutrients.

Follow-Up Treatment

Three weeks later, Mr. and Mrs. Johnson reported that since they had started to offer Lucas only his favorite foods, he was less anxious during meals but continued to get up from his chair after he had eaten for only a few minutes. He also did not like the enriched formula they tried to give him, and they had to experiment with different flavors until he decided that he liked the chocolate-flavored one the best. He liked to drink his formula from the bottle instead of a cup and could not go to sleep without his bottle, although he was drinking water and juice from a regular cup during the day.

After receiving this interim information, I discussed with the parents how we should prioritize the different aspects of Lucas's treatment. Because Lucas was not able to go to sleep without his bottle and had just made the transition to the enriched formula, we agreed that we would not try to wean him off the bottle at this point of the treatment. We also discussed how to make him feel hungry and learn to eat until fullness as the next step of treatment.

To help Lucus learn to feel his hunger and eat until fullness, I worked with his parents to institute the feeding guidelines. The parents worked out a schedule of regular meals at 3- to 4-hour intervals, and Mr. Johnson agreed to be home for the family dinner at 6:30 p.m. Lucas was not to drink from the bottle or snack in any way between these regular meals and the scheduled afternoon snack. He could only drink water in between meals and the afternoon snack in order to make him hungry at mealtimes.

At mealtime, he had to sit at the table until "Mommy's and Daddy's tummies were full." The parents were to give him small portions of his favorite foods, and he could have second, third, and fourth helpings until his tummy was full. This way he was going to be less likely to be overwhelmed by the food and learn to recognize the feeling of fullness. If he were to throw food or get up from the table before the parents had finished eating, he was going to get one warning and then go in time-out. *(The time-out procedure is described in detail in the chapter on Infantile Anorexia. The emphasis is on the child's learning to accept limits, to calm himself, and to correct his behavior.)* I explained that these feeding guidelines were primarily geared to treat the Infantile Anorexia, to help Lucas become more aware of his feelings of hunger and fullness, and to bring some structure into their lives.

As far as the Sensory Food Aversions were concerned, I reemphasized that the best they could do at this point was to relax, because they were able to give Lucas the essential nutrients through the enriched formula, and they should wait until he was ready to venture into trying new foods.

At the end of the 2-hour session, Mr. and Mrs. Johnson expressed feelings of relief because they understood Lucas better, and they felt that they had a plan on how to help him.

The next appointment was 3 weeks later and included my observation of a family meal from behind the mirror. During the meal, Lucas stayed in his chair and seemed more relaxed eating his hot dog and french fries, which had become his daily staples. After about 5 minutes of eating, he paused and noticed the microphone on the ceiling. However, his parents were able to redirect him to continue eating by giving him a small portion of pudding. He continued to be distractible throughout the meal, but each time he made comments on what he saw in the room, his parents confirmed his observations and then redirected him to his food. There was no throwing of food and no effort by Lucas to get out of his chair. When Lucas stopped eating and did not want any more food, Mrs. Johnson asked him whether his tummy was full and Lucas said yes. Mrs. Johnson replied that he had to wait until Mommy's and Daddy's tummies were full, and after a few minutes, Lucas started to eat again for another 10 minutes. *(I have made the observation with a number of children with Infantile Anorexia that they state that their tummy is full but continue to eat if they have to sit at the table and wait for their parents to finish with their meal. It appears to me that when the edge is taken off their hunger, they interpret this to be full, and if allowed, they will terminate the meal. However, if they have to stay at the table and there is nothing else for them to do or to entertain themselves, they continue eating for another 10 or 15 minutes until they are really full. This is very important because I have learned that children with Infantile Anorexia not only have difficulty recognizing hunger, but they also seem not to know when they are full, and they tend to stop eating as soon as the edge is taken off their weak hunger feelings.)*

After the meal, I met with Mr. and Mrs. Johnson to discuss how things had been going since our last meeting. They reported that Lucas got his first time-out for getting up from the table during the meal and that he cried for more than half an hour until he finally calmed himself. However, when he returned to the table, he sat quietly for a few minutes, then started to eat some pretzels and sat at the table until his parents stopped eating and asked him whether his tummy was full. After this rather long first time-out, Lucas accepted that he had to stay at the table, and he had not challenged his parents about this anymore. *Because sitting at the table during mealtimes is so important for any child with a feeding disorder, I encourage parents to make sure that when the child returns to the table after the time-out that they eat for another 5 minutes and that the child sits at the table with them regardless of how long the child has been in time-out and regardless of whether the child eats or not. This way the child realizes that the parents are not making him eat but rather requiring that he sit with them until they are finished with the meal. Interestingly, most children like Lucas need only one time-out in order to accept that they have to sit at the table until "Mommy and Daddy's tummies are full."*

The parents reported that since they had introduced the feeding guidelines, Lucas ate more at most meals but continued to have some meals when he ate very little. Although Mr. and Mrs. Johnson were still paying close attention to how much or how little Lucas ate, they professed that they had done away with all distractions during mealtime and had stopped making comments about the amount of food Lucas ate. They felt that Lucas was watching carefully what they were eating, but he had not shown any interest in trying their food. Overall, they felt that things were getting better but seemed disappointed that Lucas had not asked for any of their foods. I explained to the parents that most children do not recover from the past experiences of having to try new foods so quickly and usually take months until they seem relaxed enough to put a new food in their mouth.

Mr. and Mrs. Johnson wanted to continue with the present arrangement for another month and come back to work on getting Lucas off the bottle. In the meantime, I encouraged them to offer Lucas some of the enriched formula out of a cup at each mealtime.

During the next appointment I saw Mr. and Mrs. Johnson without Lucas. They were pleased that Lucas was getting more focused and more relaxed during mealtime and that he had expressed feeling hungry a few times before dinner. Overall, he was eating more, but he continued to stick to his limited diet, eating no vegetables, no fruits, and no meats except hot dogs. He still had not asked to try any new food. He had started to accept some enriched formula during mealtimes but continued to ask for his bottle before his nap and at bedtime. The parents had to use time-out for some misbehavior unrelated to mealtimes and felt that Lucas was usually able to calm himself within a few minutes. When Lucas recently saw his pediatrician, he had gained some weight and grown an inch, which was very encouraging to the parents.

Considering the good news about Lucas's increased appetite, his improved growth, his willingness to drink some enriched formula out of the cup, and his improved ability to calm himself, I encouraged the parents to wean him off the bottle. Because Lucas did not know how to put himself to sleep without the bottle, I helped the parents develop a sleep routine of first staying with him until Lucas was asleep and then gradually fading out. In order to compensate for the loss of calories and micronutrients, I suggested that they offer Lucas enriched formula with each meal.

During the following appointment, a month later, I saw the whole family again. Lucas had been weaned off the bottle, had started to attend pre-school 3 days a week, and had eaten some of the food that they offered at lunch time at school, which he had never eaten before. On my advice, the parents had talked to the teacher about his Sensory Food Aversions and asked the teacher not to force Lucas to eat any of the food they offered at school if he did not want to eat it. However, when Lucas saw the other children enjoying the food, he seemed to get encouraged to eat it as well.

During the lunch meal at the hospital, Lucas looked relaxed and enjoyed his hot dog and french fries, which continued to be his "safe foods," but he showed some interest in the watermelon his parents were eating and asked to have a piece. He tried it and did not seem to be sure whether he liked it, and he did not ask for any more. He was less distractible and stayed in his chair for the entire meal.

The parents seemed relieved that Lucas was making progress with being more aware of his hunger and fullness feelings and that he was starting to get interested in trying new foods, mostly at school but also some at home. They felt that since he had given up the bottle feedings, his appetite had improved and he had shown more interest in new foods. He was drinking enriched formula at each meal, and we decided that they would continue this because his diet was still rather limited and missing some of the essential micronutrients, especially vitamins.

Final Outcome

This was the last regular visit by Lucas and his family. I told Lucas and his parents that when he was older and wanted to learn to eat more new foods but was scared to do so, he should tell his parents and I could help him how to do that.

Lucas came back when he was 8 years old. He was a tall slender boy and seemed to be well regulated with his eating. He had expanded his diet somewhat over the years, but it bothered him that his friends were eating pizza, hamburgers, and apples, and he was afraid to try them. He worked with me on getting the courage to eat these foods one bite at a time, and within a year, he had expanded his diet and begun enjoying most of the foods his friends were eating.

Complex Feeding Disorders

As pointed out previously, children can have more than one feeding disorder. They can develop two feeding disorders at the same time, such as Infantile Anorexia and Sensory Food Aversions, which both commonly start during the first 3 years of life, as I have described in the case above. However, they can also develop one feeding disorder first and then develop another one on top of it as they grow older. In my clinical experience, this often happens with young infants who suffer from gastroesophageal reflux. They start out refusing to continue feeding when they experience distress, which is often after they have taken in 1 or 2 ounces of milk. They may return to feeding when the distress subsides and stop again when they become distressed. If this is recognized as a Feeding Disorder Associated With a Concurrent Medical Condition, and the underlying gastroesophageal reflux is treated effectively, the feeding disorder may resolve, and the infant may outgrow the gastroesophageal reflux and be fine. However, if the infant is very sensitive to pain and makes an association between feeding and distress, the infant may become fearful to feed and may develop a Posttraumatic Feeding Disorder. The infant will become distressed at the sight of the bottle when positioned for feeding and will refuse to drink from the bottle altogether (see the case of Vivian in the chapter on Posttraumatic Feeding Disorder).

It is very important to take a good history of the child's feeding development, to sort out what may underlie the child's feeding difficulties, and to recognize that the child may have several feeding disorders that compound the feeding problems. Once the different feeding disorders have been identified, the clinician needs to develop a plan how to prioritize the treatment of the child.

The following case illustrates the complexity of understanding and treating a child who had four feeding disorders. He started out with a Feeding Disorder Associated With a Concurrent Medical Condition (gastroesophageal reflux and a metabolic disorder), then developed symptoms of Infantile Anorexia and Sensory Food Aversions, and during the treatment in another facility developed a Posttraumatic Feeding Disorder. I will begin with the presenting symptoms from a letter that the child's desperate mother sent to a nurse practitioner at our facility where the child had been treated earlier for his rare metabolic disorder. Like I have done with all case histories, I have changed the names and some of the details of the history to protect the identity of the child and his family. I will indicate in parentheses which symptoms are characteristic of which feeding disorder, and I will comment on the symptoms and their treatment as I go along with the description of the case.

Example 2

Chief Complaints

The mother, Mrs. Green, wrote: Rolf is now 18 months old and overall doing very well. He is developing normally, is very energetic and an incredibly engaging and happy child. However, since about 8 months, we have been wrestling constantly with feeding issues. He has been really hard to feed: a picky eater with a quick gag *(symptoms of Sensory Food Aversions)* and no demonstrable desire to eat *(symptom of Infantile Anorexia)*.

We found over time that the best way to get food in him was extravagant distractions, though it did not always keep the food down. Rolf has a habit of vomiting, sometimes a few times in a day, and sometimes not for weeks *(the vomiting could have been triggered by Sensory Food Aversions or by gastro-esophageal reflux)*. It has made mealtime really, really stressful. He has never seemed to be in any sort of pain or discomfort, and often appears to "choose" to vomit at particular times that we can predict. He has definite behavioral ties to some instances of emeses, but other times they are rather out-of-the-blue. *(It is not clear what Mrs. Green means by the "behavioral ties" of Rolf's vomiting, that Rolf "'chooses' to vomit at particular times." However, the vomiting in response to an aversive food is often interpreted by parents as willful. The unpredictable "out-of-the-blue" vomiting could be explained by gastroesophageal reflux.)*

Things escalated since he reached 12 months and we have been trying to get him over to table foods and some self-feeding. Meals were taking incredibly long, and his vomiting was slowing down the process of getting calories into him. I was spending an average of 6 or 7 hours a day feeding him … in front of the television, Elmo to be precise. It was killing me. *(Resorting to all kind of distractions is often described by parents of toddlers who have Infantile Anorexia and are not interested in feeding.)*

We talked to our pediatrician, who figured that it was time we got some help from a feeding program. He always wrote off the vomiting as "happy regurgitation" and suggested it was a vestigial remnant of his gaggy past, and something that he might grow out of or we could find ways to work around. But perhaps we needed some therapy or at least a good assessment of his feeding "disorder," because he just didn't seem to want to eat.

He suggested that we go down to the feeding clinic closest to us, and we were set up with a therapy program we have been going to twice a week for a few weeks now. They have us perform an elaborate circus every mealtime, with television, toys, bubbles, timers, and all sorts of routines. I know that these are designed to be helpful, but since we started the "method," Rolf's vomiting has really increased. Now it is impossible to get a meal into him without at least one incident of emesis. Last weekend, he threw up 17 times.

The vomiting comes in different forms. Sometimes, it is a classic gag. Sometimes, he will throw up if he does not like the taste of something *(both are symptoms of Sensory Food Aversions).* Currently, he will throw up almost every time that I approach him with a spoon, and he gags at the sound of the baby jar opening sometimes *(symptoms of Posttraumatic Feeding Disorder).* Once he is out of the high chair, he is completely fine. He never throws up when he is not in the high chair. If he grabs something to munch on while he is playing in the living room, he won't gag or vomit.

Past Feeding and Medical History

As I have indicated in my comments in parentheses, Mrs. Green gives a very clear description of the different feeding difficulties of Rolf. In order to understand his problems more fully, I elicited the following feeding and medical history:

Rolf was born full-term but would not nurse except for one or two short instances. He was admitted to a local hospital to the neonatal intensive care unit and fed breast milk through a nasogastric tube. After 10 days, he was transferred to our tertiary care center, where he was diagnosed with severe gastroesophageal reflux disease. He received occupational therapy for what was considered an "oral aversion" and continued to vomit quite frequently throughout his 20-day inpatient treatment. He was discharged on nasogastric tube-feedings, and after 5 days readmitted to the hospital after he started to vomit blood. Because of severe gastritis also in the pyloric channel, the nasogastric tube was replaced by a naso-jejunal tube, and an occupational therapist worked with Rolf to help him with oral feedings. However, the vomiting continued until the feeding tube was removed and Rolf underwent surgery to place a Broviac catheter for total parenteral nutrition. Rolf started to take small amounts of food by bottle and accepted the pacifier. A rare metabolic disease was diagnosed, and Rolf received biweekly injections to correct the metabolic defect. After 2 months in the hospital, he was discharged home, drinking some milk from the bottle but receiving most of his nutrition parenterally.

Rolf gradually began to take more nutrition by mouth, and 6 weeks later, a follow-up examination showed complete resolution of the gastritis. When he began to take adequate nutrition by mouth a few weeks later, the Broviac catheter was removed. The parents were trained to continue the twice weekly injections for treatment of his metabolic disease, and Rolf became healthy and developed normally.

By 6 months of age, Rolf was introduced to baby food, but he showed little interest in feeding. Mrs. Green had hoped that going to solid foods and then to table food would spark Rolf's interest in food, but she found herself going to elaborate lengths to get meals into him as he grew older. *(This is a typical way parents describe children who have a low hunger drive as seen in Infantile Anorexia. As the infants get older and learn to crawl and then walk, it seems that there are so many interesting things to explore and to learn that eating becomes "boring," as older children with Infantile Anorexia have told me. Because of the children's curiosity and their interest in everything else but food, the parents find themselves using toys and television to entertain them, while they feed them.)*

With the introduction of various baby foods and solid foods, Rolf started to vomit again. Mrs. Green recalled that when she fed him applesauce, bananas, green beans, and potatoes, he spit the food out, sometimes gagged, and then vomited everything up. When she offered these foods again, Rolf refused to open his mouth, pushed the food away, and cried if she did not remove these foods. This happened with several other foods, and the list of foods Rolf would be willing to accept became shorter and shorter. *(Rolf's aversive reactions to certain foods, which ranged from grimacing and spitting out the food to gagging and vomiting, are typical of Sensory Food Aversions. Following these aversive reactions, most children refuse to continue eating the aversive foods and may refuse other foods that they have never tried.)*

So far Mrs. Green has described Rolf's early symptoms of gastroesophageal reflux with severe gastritis, which was successfully treated, and Rolf was symptom-free for a while until the vomiting recurred, when he was introduced to a variety of baby foods and table foods that were aversive to him. I have observed that children with a history of gastroesophageal reflux are more prone to not only gag but also vomit if they eat a food that triggers an aversive reaction. In addition, Mrs. Green had become concerned about Rolf's little interest in food and her having to use all kinds of distractions in order to get him to eat. In summary, by the time he was 1 year old, Rolf had developed symptoms of Infantile Anorexia, Sensory Food Aversions, and reactivation of his gastroesophageal reflux.

Because feedings became increasingly stressful and took 6 to 7 hours a day, Mrs. Green had asked her pediatrician for help. In the letter to the nurse practitioner at our hospital, whom Mrs. Green had gotten to know during Rolf's early hospitalization, she explained that the pediatrician had referred Rolf to a feeding disorders program closest to where the family lived. During the twice weekly therapy visits, Mrs. Green was taught to use positive reinforcement for every bite of food Rolf would accept through giving him toys, videos, and praise. She was asked to stop allowing him to feed himself, which he had been doing some during each meal before. However, after a few days on the recommended regimen, Rolf began to vomit profusely. Whereas before he had vomited 2–3 times a week, he began vomiting 2–3 times a meal, and according to the instructions by the therapists in the program, Mrs. Green had refed him the emesis after each vomiting as negative reinforcement of his vomiting.

As Mrs. Green described in the letter above, Rolf started to gag and vomit at the sound of his mother's opening of the baby jars or her approaching him with the spoon. These are classic signs of a Posttraumatic Feeding Disorder. Not only was Rolf traumatized by his mother's refeeding him the emesis, but Mrs. Green also was terrified that Rolf was going to die because of all the vomiting that followed. Because Rolf's vomiting was interpreted as behavioral, the negative reinforcement was supposed to stop the vomiting but had done just the opposite and traumatized mother and child.

What this case illustrates very clearly is that there is no *place in the treatment of feeding disorders for "refeeding the emesis to a child." I have talked to older children who had been in similar behavioral treatment programs and had been subjected to refeeding of their emesis. These children were all traumatized by the experience. They described their feelings of helplessness, of not being able to control their vomiting, and the rage they experienced when they were punished for their vomiting. They had become distrustful of professionals who were supposed to help them, and it was difficult for them to overcome their fears and to establish a therapeutic relationship with other professionals. In addition, not only were the children traumatized by their experience, but the parents were traumatized and enraged as well. In each of these cases the vomiting was caused by Sensory Food Aversions or by organic problems, but was interpreted by the professionals as "behavioral" and purposeful by the child.*

After vomiting 17 times on a weekend, the feeding program suspected some medical reason for the vomiting and recommended more medical tests by gastroenterology. Rolf underwent several tests that confirmed gastroesophageal reflux. The gastroenterologist recommended a more relaxed feeding program and treated the gastroesophageal reflux with medication. The parents discontinued the relationship with the feeding program. They decided to stop refeeding Rolf the meals if he vomited and to allow him to feed himself the last meal of the day when eating with the family at the table. The vomiting decreased to about once a day. However, the parents noted that Rolf began gagging if he saw food that he did not like, or if he got bored with the video he was watching while the parents fed him.

The treatment of the gastroesophageal reflux and no longer refeeding Rolf his emesis seemed to decrease the vomiting. However, Rolf continued to show anticipatory fear and gagging when he saw foods that he did not like, foods that had caused him gagging and vomiting in the past. I have observed in several children who had Sensory Food Aversions and who had been force-fed by their parents or by therapists that they developed a Posttraumatic Feeding Disorder. The children, just like Rolf, would become so frightened of having to eat aversive foods that they would gag and vomit at the sight of food. The gagging and vomiting are often misinterpreted as "willful" and oppositional, and the children are punished for something they cannot control.

The Observation of Feeding and Play

Rolf was a delightful and outgoing little boy of 18 months who was engaged with both of his parents and enjoyed playing with the cars and blocks. However, when it came to going into the high chair, he started to cry and did not want to sit down until his mother started to play the television. He appeared mesmerized by the television, and if his mother caught him at a moment when he seemed completely absorbed by the television, she was able to put the spoon in his mouth. After having fed him a jar of baby food, she offered him some Cheerios, which he fed himself without taking his eyes off the television screen. The moment the father turned off the television, Rolf stopped feeding himself and struggled to get out of the high chair. There was no vomiting during or after the feeding.

The observation of the feeding revealed that Rolf continued to be fearful of feeding but could be distracted by the television and that the relationship between Rolf and his parents had not been affected by the traumatic feeding experiences of the past.

The Nutritional Assessment

Despite all the feeding difficulties, Rolf had grown along the 25th percentile for height and weight and the 50th percentile for head circumference. He looked well-nourished and healthy. His mother's heroic efforts to feed him for 6 to 7 hours daily had put him in an excellent nutritional range.

Summary and Interpretation of the Findings

At the time of the evaluation, Rolf presented with four feeding disorders. As a newborn, Rolf had shown feeding resistance that was believed to be caused by severe gastritis, gastroesophageal reflux, and a rare metabolic disorder. He was successfully treated and symptom-free when he was about 5 to 6 months old. However, with the introduction of various baby foods and later table foods, Rolf experienced aversive reactions to a number of foods. These reactions ranged from grimacing and spitting out the food to gagging and vomiting. After these aversive reactions, Rolf refused to eat these foods anymore and started to refuse most of the other foods that his mother offered him. He preferred to feed himself Cheerios, which he tolerated well. In addition, the vomiting caused by the Sensory Food Aversions reactivated his gastroesophageal reflux, and Rolf started to vomit at other times without provocation.

In addition, when Rolf became mobile and learned to sit up and move about, he showed no interest in feeding. His mother noticed that if she distracted him, she could slip the spoon into his mouth without him protesting it. As Rolf got older, she found herself more and more challenged in coming up with distractions that would allow her to feed him, and she spent 6 to 7 hours daily trying to get food into him. This is a classic story of a child with Infantile Anorexia. Children with Infantile Anorexia show little or no hunger signals, especially when they learn to move around and their little world becomes more and more interesting. Parents like Mrs. Green find themselves trapped in regulating their children's food intake by distracting them during feedings for hours on end.

Finally, when the parents turned for help to a feeding program, Rolf was treated with positive and negative reinforcers for each bite of food that he accepted or refused. The negative reinforcers included refeeding him the emesis if he vomited. The mother, Mrs. Green, was trained to use these techniques at home. There was no recognition that Rolf's vomiting was triggered by Sensory Food

Aversions and that he could not control it. Consequently, Rolf became very frightened of being fed and started to gag and vomit in anticipation of feedings, when his mother opened the baby jar or approached him with the spoon. Rolf developed a Posttraumatic Feeding Disorder characterized by anticipatory anxiety and refusal to be fed. When the parents realized what was happening, they discontinued the treatment, but Rolf continued to be frightened to go into the high chair and resisted feedings.

Despite all these feeding difficulties, Mrs. Green had managed to get enough food into Rolf, and he was physically healthy and well nourished. However, both mother and child were very traumatized by their feeding experience.

Treatment

Initial Recommendations

The first step of the treatment consisted of helping the parents understand the components of the four different feeding disorders that I have outlined above. With the help of a handout for each feeding disorder, I explained to the parents Rolf's feeding history and helped them understand his fear of feedings and his food refusal. Then I discussed with them that we needed to prioritize how we could help Rolf to learn to feed without fear and eventually regulate his eating internally instead of the parents having to work on every spoonful going in his mouth.

Because Mrs. Green was in the last month of pregnancy and was frightened that Rolf would not live if she did not get enough food into him, the parents decided that Mr. Green was going to take a month off from work and take over Rolf's feeding. To prevent any more aversive reactions, I asked Mrs. Green to make a list of foods that had led to Rolf's spitting out the food, gagging, or vomiting, and I asked the parents not to offer Rolf any of those foods anymore unless he asked to have some.

Both parents were very concerned about how to get food into Rolf, and Mr. Green felt that if he distracted Rolf with television, wrapped him in a blanket, and held him on his lap, he was able to feed him without a struggle. I advised the parents to have Rolf have one meal at dinner in the high chair, while the parents were eating their own dinner, in order to get Rolf back into feeding himself. I encouraged them to present Rolf with toys while sitting in the high chair to break the association of the high chair and vomiting. Once Rolf was comfortable in the high chair, I asked the parents to remove the toys and to offer Rolf Cheerios and other snack foods that he had eaten before when they were left out. I emphasized that the meal in the high chair was not meant to get calories into Rolf, but should allow him to learn to relax during meals and feed himself.

Follow-Up Appointments

Three weeks later, Mr. Green returned with Rolf alone, because Mrs. Green had delivered a baby girl 9 days before. Mr. Green reported that he had fed Rolf as we had discussed. He had wrapped him in a blanket, and Rolf accepted the feedings without struggle, but Mr. Green was concerned that Rolf continued to vomit after almost every meal except when he fed himself in the high chair. When I observed the feeding, Rolf went into the high chair without protest, but was very distractible, played with the food, and threw it off the tray rather than putting any in his mouth.

I suggested to Mr. Green that he offer Rolf only two Cheerios at a time, model for him how to chew, and wait until Rolf had swallowed the Cheerios before giving him any more. I have found this to be an effective way to keep toddlers with Infantile Anorexia involved with eating and engaged with their parents in a nonconflictual way. I discussed with Mr. Green whether he might overfeed Rolf during the "television feedings" and trigger more reflux, but I also referred him back to gastroenterology to see whether Rolf's medication needed to be adjusted.

A few weeks later, both parents and the baby accompanied Rolf for his appointment. Rolf's medication had been increased and Mr. Green had cut back some on the amount of food during the "television feedings." Rolf had vomited only occasionally, and the feedings in the high chair had gone better when he started to give Rolf only a few pieces of food at a time. However, when I observed the meal, Mr. Green used a lot of exaggerated modeling of chewing and swallowing to keep Rolf interested in the feeding.

When I suggested that Mr. Green decrease the television feedings to twice daily and have Rolf feed himself the other two meals, both parents became very anxious and expressed concern that Rolf would not get enough calories. It became clear to me that they were not ready to make that move. Consequently, I suggested that I weigh and measure Rolf during each visit, so that we could monitor his growth while allowing him to take over more meals.

During the next visit, a month later, the parents reported that they had gone down to two television feedings, one in the morning and one in the evening. Mr. Green had gone back to work, and Mrs. Green had taken over these feedings. She reported that she did not have to wrap Rolf in the blanket anymore, and that he did not resist her feeding him as long as he was watching television. The two other meals when he was self-feeding were inconsistent. Sometimes he ate quite well, but other times he was very distractible and ate very little. The parents took comfort from knowing that Rolf had gained a little weight since the last visit and agreed to give up another television feeding.

The following month, the parents were ready to give up all the television feedings but needed another month until Mr. Green was able to give up the exaggerated modeling of chewing and swallowing when Rolf was feeding himself. At that time, I introduced the parents to the feeding guidelines and the time-out procedure (described in detail in the chapter on Infantile Anorexia).

In the meantime, Rolf had grown into a 2-year-old toddler who wanted to assert himself and had figured that he could exercise control over his parents by not eating. The parents were gradually able to relax and not panic if he ate little to nothing during a meal, and they began to develop increasing confidence that Rolf could regulate his eating internally. He continued to gain weight at a normal rate and became a muscular little boy.

However, he continued to be very selective about what foods he was willing to put in his mouth. He refused all "slippery" foods, but gradually started to ask to try some of the more crunchy foods he observed his parents eating. He drank an enriched formula that provided him with all the necessary nutrients and that allowed his parents to relax and wait for him to decide which foods he was willing to try.

After 10 months of treatment, the family moved away, confident that their little boy was on the way to healthy eating. A year later, I received a Christmas card showing a happy family, with greetings and thanks from the parents for helping them to have confidence in Rolf that he could regulate his eating internally.

I hope that through this case, I have been able to illustrate the importance of the diagnostic assessment and the significance of understanding the different feeding disorders in order to choose the appropriate treatment.

References

Chatoor, I. & Ammaniti, M. (2007). A classification of feeding disorders of infancy and early childhood. In W. Narrow, M. First, P. Sirovatka, & D. Reiger (Eds.), *Age and Gender Considerations in Psychiatric Diagnosis: A Research Agenda for DSM-V* (pp. 227–242). Arlington, VA: American Psychiatric Press Inc.

Chatoor, I. Ganiban, J., Macaoay, M., Harrison, J., Kerzner, B., McWade-Paez, et al. (2007, October). "A classification of feeding disorders in infants and young children: clinical presentation and diagnostic inter-rater agreement". In *Scientific Program and Abstracts*, Eating Disorders Research Society, Pittsburgh, PA, October 25–27, 2007, p. 45.

Narrow, W. E., First, M. B., Sirovatka, P., & Regier, D. A. (Eds.). (2007). *Age and gender considerations in psychiatric diagnosis: A research agenda for DSM-V*. Arlington, VA: American Psychiatric Press.

PARENT INFORMATION OUTLINE

Irene Chatoor, MD

INFANTILE ANOREXIA

Description:

- The central problem for children with Infantile Anorexia is their lack of appetite ("anorexia"), which leads to disinterest in feeding and to food refusal.

- Infantile Anorexia is quite different from the commonly known Anorexia Nervosa, in which the individuals have an intense fear of gaining weight, which results in a purposeful restriction of their food intake.

- The onset is before 3 years of age, most commonly between 9 and 18 months, when the world gets more interesting, and the child is transitioned to spoon- and self-feeding.

- Children with Infantile Anorexia rarely show any signals of hunger, which causes most parents to become worried and anxious because it puts the burden on them to get their children to eat.

- Often, these children take only a few bites before they refuse to eat any more. The few bites they do take seem just enough to take the edge off any hunger they may experience, and they do not eat until fullness.

- Once the edge is taken off, the children may throw feeding utensils and food and frequently try to climb out of the high chair or leave the table to play. These children are more interested in their surroundings, and they would rather play and interact with their caregivers than eat.

- Because parents are often worried about their children's poor growth, they feel they need to coax, distract, threaten, and entertain to get their children to eat. Sometimes they may even force their children to eat during mealtimes. These methods may work initially; however, they are not a long-term solution. In fact, the more these behaviors go on during mealtime, the more the children become completely unaware of hunger, and their food intake becomes externally regulated by their parents.

PARENT INFORMATION OUTLINE

Irene Chatoor, MD

SENSORY FOOD AVERSIONS

Description:

- Children with Sensory Food Aversions consistently refuse to eat certain foods and the refusal is related to the taste, texture, smell, temperature, and/or appearance of the food. This is different from children refusing to eat a particular food one day but eating it the next.

- Food aversions are common and believed to occur along a spectrum of severity, with some children refusing only a few specific foods and others refusing whole food groups (e.g., vegetables, fruits, or meats).

- Reactions to the aversive foods can range from grimacing to more severe reactions such as gagging, vomiting, or spitting out the food.

- After they experience the initial aversive reaction, children with Sensory Food Aversions usually refuse to continue eating that particular food and become very distressed if forced to do so.

- In fact, after an aversive experience, some children tend to generalize and refuse foods that look and/or smell like the aversive food (e.g., an aversion to peas may be generalized to all green foods).

- Children with Sensory Food Aversions will eat well if given the foods they prefer.

- Oftentimes parents report that these children are reluctant to try new foods.

- Some children are so sensitive that they will refuse to eat any foods that have touched other foods on their plates, while others eat only foods of specific brand names or restaurants (e.g., will only eat McDonald's chicken nuggets).

- If these children refuse whole food groups, their diet may become deficient in vitamins, minerals (e.g., zinc or iron), or protein.

Continued

- If these children reject foods that require significant chewing (e.g., meats or hard vegetables), they fall behind in their oral motor development due to lack of experience/practice with chewing, and they may have articulation problems.

- Food sensitivities may extend to aversions in other sensory areas (e.g., touching certain foods, walking on sand or grass, the feeling of clothing labels, loud noises and bright lights).

Irene Chatoor, MD

POSTTRAUMATIC FEEDING DISORDER

Description:

- Children with Posttraumatic Feeding Disorder display fear and intense resistance to either eating solid food or drinking from the bottle. In more severe cases, they may refuse to eat or drink altogether.

- Some parents report that the child's refusal to eat any solid foods or drink from the bottle followed an incidence of choking, gagging, vomiting, or force–feeding.

- Some parents report that the child's food refusal followed the insertion of feeding tubes, intubation, or major surgery that required vigorous oropharyngeal suctioning.

- Reminders of the traumatic events (e.g., bottle, bib, or high chair) frequently cause intense distress, which may lead to fearful reactions from the child when positioned for feedings and presented with feeding utensils and food. These reminders sometimes even lead to gagging and vomiting.

- Children with Posttraumatic Feeding Disorder resist being fed by crying, arching, and refusing to open their mouths.

- If food is placed in the child's mouth, he will intensely resist swallowing. The child may actively spit the food out or store the food in his cheeks and spit it out later.

- In children with Posttraumatic Feeding Disorder, the fear of eating seems to override any awareness of hunger.

- Children with Posttraumatic Feeding Disorder who refuse all foods and liquids require acute intervention to prevent dehydration and starvation.

Irene Chatoor, MD

FEEDING DISORDER ASSOCIATED WITH A CONCURRENT MEDICAL CONDITION

Description:

- The child usually initiates feeding without difficulty and may eat or drink an ounce or two.

- However, while feeding, the child may experience distress, cry, and push the bottle or food away.

- The child may be so distressed that he or she refuses to resume feeding.

- The child has a concurrent medical condition (e.g., reflux, allergic gastritis, heart or lung disease) that is believed to cause the distress.

- The child's food intake is inadequate for growth.

- The child may fail to gain weight or may lose weight.

ABOUT THE AUTHOR

IRENE CHATOOR, MD

Dr. Chatoor is vice chair of the Department of Psychiatry and Behavioral Sciences and director of the Infant and Toddler Mental Health Program at Children's National Medical Center, as well as professor of Psychiatry and Pediatrics at the George Washington University School of Medicine in Washington, DC. Her research on early childhood feeding disorders, with a special focus on the diagnosis and treatment of Infantile Anorexia, has been funded through the National Institute of Mental Health and a grant from the National Center for Research Resources awarded to Children's Research Institute. She is the author of more than 50 papers and several book chapters. Dr. Chatoor has presented her research findings at national and international conferences and has been invited internationally to train professionals in the diagnosis and treatment of feeding disorders.